NATIONAL INSTITUTE SOCIAL SERVICES LIBRARY

Volume

T0256222

SOCIAL WORK AND
SOCIAL VALUES

SOCIAL WORK AND SOCIAL VALUES

Readings in Social Work, Volume 3

Edited by
EILEEN YOUNGHUSBAND

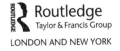

Routledge
Taylor & Francis Group

LONDON AND NEW YORK

First published in 1967 by George Allen & Unwin Ltd.

This edition first published in 2022
by Routledge
4 Park Square, Milton Park, Abingdon, Oxon OX14 4RN
605 Third Avenue, New York, NY 10017

Routledge is an imprint of the Taylor & Francis Group, an informa business

© 1967 by Taylor & Francis.

British Library Cataloguing in Publication Data
A catalogue record for this book is available from the British Library

ISBN: 978-1-03-203381-5 (Set)
ISBN: 978-1-00-321681-0 (Set) (ebk)
ISBN: 978-1-03-205944-0 (Volume 41) (hbk)
ISBN: 978-1-03-205946-4 (Volume 41) (pbk)
ISBN: 978-1-00-319999-1 (Volume 41) (ebk)

DOI: 10.4324/9781003199991

Publisher's Note
The publisher has gone to great lengths to ensure the quality of this reprint but points out that some imperfections in the original copies may be apparent.

Disclaimer
The publisher has made every effort to trace copyright holders and would welcome correspondence from those they have been unable to trace.

SOCIAL WORK
AND
SOCIAL VALUES

READINGS IN SOCIAL WORK

VOLUME III

COMPILED BY

EILEEN YOUNGHUSBAND

D.B.E., LL.D.

London
GEORGE ALLEN & UNWIN LTD
RUSKIN HOUSE · MUSEUM STREET

FIRST PUBLISHED IN 1967

SECOND IMPRESSION 1970

© George Allen & Unwin Ltd, 1967

SBN 04 361008 0

PRINTED IN GREAT BRITAIN

BY PHOTOLITHOGRAPHY

BY COMPTON PRINTING LTD.

LONDON AND AYLESBURY

PREFACE

This volume is the third in a series intended to preserve in more permanent form some of the most valuable articles which have appeared in British and American social work journals in the last few years. There are certain articles which are widely used and quoted, which have indeed become standard works but are not always easily available to busy social workers. The aim of the present series is thus twofold, both to preserve such articles and make them more widely available and at the same time to combine together the best that has been written on a given theme by social workers on both sides of the Atlantic which draw attention to recent developments in thought and knowledge.

The present volume includes articles which are directly concerned with cultural and ethical values, or with increased understanding of people whose behaviour is pathological, in relation to western value systems. It also contains articles on the relation between an administrative structure and professional goals. It concludes with four articles which give particularly sensitive accounts of social work with people under acute stress, and which thus illustrate in action social work's concern for those suffering from deprivation and conflict, whether as would-be adoptive or foster parents or in the face of illness and death.

It is hoped that this collection of articles will be widely used by practising social workers, by social work teachers and by students not only in Great Britain and the United States but in those many other parts of the world where the profession of social work is advancing towards higher standards of practice.

The National Institute for Social Work Training has received much helpful co-operation from the authors of the articles which form this book and from the journals in which they appeared. In addition to expressing our indebtedness to the authors, the following acknowledgements are made with gratitude to the journals in which the articles originally appeared: *The Almoner* (London) for permission to reprint 'The Social Worker in the Sixties'; 'Some Thoughts about Dying' and 'Communication with the Patient'; *The British Journal of Psychiatric Social Work* published by the Association of Psychiatric Social Workers, London, for permission to reprint 'Ethics and the Social Worker'; *Case Conference*, London, for permission to reprint 'Casework and Agency Function' and 'Co-ordination Reviewed'; *Social Casework*, New York, for permission to reprint 'Family Diagnosis Variations in the Basic Values of Family Systems' and 'Ego Deficiency in Delinquents', with the permission of the Family Service Association of America, New York; *The Social Service Review* published by the University of Chicago Press, Chicago, Illinois, for permission to reprint 'The Social Worker and his Society' (Copyright 1956 by the University of Chicago), 'Are we Creating Dependency?' and 'Understanding and Evaluating a Foster Family's Capacity to meet the Needs of an Individual Child' (both Copyright 1960 by the University of Chicago) and 'Treatment of Character Disorders: A Dilemma in Casework Culture' (Copyright 1961 by the University of Chicago); *Social Work*, New York, for permission to reprint 'A Concept of Acute Situational Disorders' and 'Interpreting Rejection to Adoptive Applicants', with the permission of The National Association of Social Workers, New York; The United Nations for permission to reprint 'Principles and Assumptions Underlying Casework Practice'.

CONTENTS

CONTENTS

1

ETHICS AND THE SOCIAL WORKER*

DOROTHY EMMET

SOCIAL workers occupy an uncomfortable but potentially creative
position where social science and psychology meet and bear on the
practical situations of human life. In these situations advice has to be
given and decisions made and, as Aristotle said in distinguishing the
practical from the theoretical sciences, 'the last step is not a proposition
but an action.' The situations in which social workers have to reach
decisions are often baffling, but they can hope that their training in
social science and psychology gives them an intelligent skill in understanding people and helping them to live in a real world.

But what about *moral* judgement? Can this also be an acquired intelligent skill, and should it be directly brought to bear on the decisions
social workers make, and on those they help their clients to make? If
we say that it can, are we not saying that social work itself has in part
at least a moral aim, and that moral persuasion and even moral pressure
may be among its methods? Yet in these days the professing of moral,
as distinct from scientific aims and still more pressing them on others,
is felt to be embarrassing, if not impertinent.

The pioneers in social work were not so embarrassed. They were
clear that there were certain standards of moral, and generally of
Christian, behaviour that ought to be upheld; that many people were
failing in these, through their own fault or through circumstances not
their own fault (though I doubt whether many would have been prepared to allow that a person's moral will could be completely defeated
by circumstances). It was the job of those more fortunately placed to
encourage the less fortunate, either by exhortation or practical help or
a mixture of both, to live up to these standards. Nowadays we have
less self-assurance. The down-grading of the expression 'doing good'
is a symptom of this. When we are told in the Authorized Version
translation of Acts x, 38 that Jesus of Nazareth 'went about doing

* Published in *The British Journal of Psychiatric Social Work*, Vol. VI, No. 4, 1962.

good', this must surely have been meant as commendatory. Benjamin Franklin mentions in his *Autobiography* (1771) how impressed he had been by a book by the New England preacher Cotton Mather entitled *Essays To Do Good.* Writing about it in 1784, he says: 'When I was a boy, I met with a book, entitled *Essays To Do Good* . . . It had been so little regarded by a former possessor, that several leaves of it were torn out; but the remainder gave me such a turn of thinking, as to have an influence on my conduct through life; for I have always set a greater value on the character of a *doer of good*, than on any other kind of reputation; and if I have been, as you seem to think, a useful citizen, the public owes the advantage of it to that book.'[1] Perhaps a reason for the contemporary down-grading of the expression is suggested in an early Victorian children's book: 'For Mary truly understood the luxury of doing good.'[2] Here 'doing good' is clearly something that ministers to self-esteem. It may also have strings attached to it, or become a vested interest. My colleague Mrs Barbara Rodgers has told me of a report of a certain home for unmarried mothers which contained the remark, 'How sad it will be if after a hundred years of service this Home has to close down for lack of girls needing help'. The image of the 'do-gooder' is not that of someone notably informed by intelligence and is a label social workers seem anxious to repudiate.

Yet if the notion of 'doing good' is under suspicion, I suspect that the nerve of social work is still a deep concern, sometimes religiously rooted, to *help* people who are in various kinds of difficulties; and there may be a sense of embarrassment, even sometimes of guilt, if one feels that this is not quite scientifically respectable.

Here I want to say quite explicitly that I see no reason to feel apologetic about a concern to help. And certainly 'help' nowadays cannot be effectively given merely by good will. Apart from the fact that effective remedies for social distresses may call for political measures, help for people's individual and personal difficulties calls for expert skills, including in our Welfare State the skill of knowing which social agencies can supply the special services needed. Thus the giving of help becomes dependent on acquiring certain kinds of expert knowledge and skill, and so is being professionalized. Does the notion of a profession itself include a notion of moral responsibility to help one's fellow men?

The view that it does has been well put by Robert Merton, Professor of Sociology at Columbia University, writing of 'the threefold

---

[1] Benjamin Franklin (edition of 1906), *The Writings of Benjamin Franklin*, Macmillan Co., New York, Vol. IX, p. 208.
[2] C. R. Attlee, *The Social Worker*, G. Bell and Sons, London, 1920, p. 9.

composite of social values that makes up the concept of a profession'. He lists these as 'first, the value placed upon systematic knowledge and the intellect: knowing. Second, the value placed upon technical skill and trained capacity: doing. And third, the value placed upon putting this conjoint knowledge and skill to work in the service of others: helping. It is these three values as fused into the concept of a profession that enlists the respect of men.'[1]

If I were pressed to hazard an opinion in the controversy over whether social workers are a profession, on the way to becoming a profession, a cluster of professions, or not a profession at all, I should say that they look like a cluster of different professions surrounded by many auxiliaries, but that they are well on the way to becoming a more unified profession. A considerable diversity of types of occupation is also found in the teaching profession. If none the less it makes sense to speak of 'the teaching profession', this is not because there is a single certified standard of training, still less because there is any single professional organization, but because there is a notion of a purpose which can be pursued at a number of different stages, all of which require a certain amount of expertise. It is not easy to define this purpose: if one were to say it was the imparting of knowledge, then kindergarten teachers and university teachers would join in rising up and saying that this is not what they are exclusively or even mainly trying to do. But presumably all members of the teaching profession are engaged in some sort of exercise which involves giving instruction to people who are in some sense *in statu pupillari*. A profession demands expertise in carrying out some broadly recognizable purpose, which, however difficult it may be to define, is not just diffuse. As the sociologists would say, it involves carrying out a role of a specific kind towards others who have their complementary roles.

Am I right in detecting a certain self-consciousness in the literature where attempts are made to define both this role of the social worker and the particular specialized knowledge it involves? Thus, in *Notes on the Ethics of Social Work*, published by the Association of Social Workers in 1953,[2] a definition emerged that 'A social worker is one who, by education, vocation and training, has fitted himself for professional employment in agencies working for the happiness and stability of the individual in the community'; and the chairman, Principal Nicholson, stated that 'The social workers' claim to professional status

[1] Robert K. Merton, *Some Thoughts on the Professions in American Society*, Brown University Papers XXXVII, Brown University, U.S.A., 1960, p. 9.
[2] Association of Social Workers, *Notes on Social Work*, London, 1953.

centres upon being a specialist in human relationships, an individual trained and disciplined in human adjustments.' At the other end of the scale, Lady Wootton simplifies the requirements of the social worker to 'good manners, ability and willingness to listen, and efficient methods of record keeping', *plus* also accurate knowledge of the workings of the social services.[1]

The difficulty seems to be to find a statement of the function of social workers which is not too diffuse, not to say grandiose, on the one hand, or too pedestrian on the other, to do justice to the real demands made upon them. To call oneself an expert in human relationships and adjustments *tout court* falls into the former pitfall. For no one (not even the psychologists) can claim just to be an expert in human relationships. There must be some particular kind of relationship in which a person can claim some special understanding: in marriage guidance or child guidance, for instance; or as a probation officer in the problems of young offenders, or as an almoner in for example the problems of the adjustments of a convalescent to family life. Undoubtedly a wise and experienced social worker can also give help in a host of personal difficulties over and above those of his or her special concern—as indeed might any wise friend who wins the confidence of someone in trouble. The problem of combining a limited and specific role with a wider kind of friendship and concern comes up in any job which involves human relationships, though it may be more difficult to evade it in social work. It is sometimes suggested that casework can be a profession in itself; but I cannot help thinking that the wealth of human experience which may be acquired in casework is best geared to some particular social service, so that the help people may be given in working out their personal and emotional troubles can grow out of some specific service or information which the caseworker is able to supply. In many instances the particular service or information is all that is required. We need not assume that there is always 'something deeper behind' a simple inquiry, for instance, about how to get a pension. But there always *may* be; and to be able to sense this, and give a person the opportunity to talk, is one of the most delicate arts in social work. Yet this is very different from setting up as an expert in human relationships in general. Some people may well seem in effect to be this, but they probably operate from a base as a family doctor or parish priest, or even keeping the little shop round the corner. If a welfare agency does not succeed in being a functional base which can be recognized as such by both parties, then a social worker

[1] Barbara Wootton, *Social Science and Social Pathology*, George Allen and Unwin, London, 1959, p. 291.

may lay herself open to the comment of the housewife who remarked: 'I wish that you ladies what have nothing to do had something better to do than come and take up the time of us ladies what have.'

Social workers, then, need to have an expert function, carried out with a sympathy which enables them to receive confidences when required. The purpose of social work must not be defined in so vague and grandiloquent a way as to cut out its specific functions, nor in so coldly matter of fact a way as to leave no room for this personal relationship. Here I come back to one of Professor Merton's requirements for a profession: 'Putting conjoint knowledge and skill to work in the service of others: helping.' To help people professionally is acceptable nowadays, in a way in which 'to do good to them' apparently is not. 'Professional help' means help within the specific field in which the person is competent. In the case of an old established profession such as medicine, this field and the end to be served—the prevention and cure of disease—is generally recognized and accepted. And there is a long tradition, going back to Hippocrates, in which thinking has gone on about the role of the doctor. This could indeed be taken as the paradigm case of a considered attempt to formulate and inculcate a professional code; for instance, the distinction between professional services and profit making: the doctor may expect his fees but must not advertise or sell his services to the highest bidder. He must respect the confidences of his patients, and must cultivate what Talcott Parsons calls 'affective neutrality'. That is to say, he may not be able to help liking some of his patients better than others, but he must not allow this to affect his treatment of them, and he must guard against any emotional involvement with a patient. These are some of the elements in the ethics of the role of the doctor; the role of the patient also has its obligations, though these are not so clearly understood and cannot be made matters of formal discipline. For instance, a patient should not do what the Americans call 'shopping around'—consulting other doctors behind the back of his own doctor without telling him that he wants a second opinion.

Some of the elements in medical professional ethics, for instance 'affective neutrality' and the respecting of confidential information,[1] would no doubt be ingredients in any code of professional behaviour, including that of social workers. But there is a special difficulty in the case of social work. In a profession such as medicine, the professional code is designed so that the doctor can properly carry out a generally

---

[1] This does not mean that there are *no* circumstances in which it would be right to divulge this.

accepted and recognized purpose. His professional ethics are therefore primarily concerned with means. But in the case of some professions, notably social work and education, the end itself is controversial and difficult to state, and any way of stating it is likely to have some ethical notion built into it, either overtly or in a concealed way. It is concealed when the end is described in terms which sound scientifically neutral, but are in fact question-begging. (When we come to think about it, do we really approve of 'harmony' and 'adjustment' in every possible kind of society? If people are being helped to 'realize their potentialities' are all potentialities desirable? If the end is 'social health', is this not really a metaphor for some state of affairs which includes morality?) Of a selection of definitions of a social worker listed in *A Report on Registration and the Social Worker*, I prefer No. 6: 'A social worker is a person who, through professional education, has acquired (1) special knowledge of the nature and needs of individuals and groups and of society; and (2) special skill in methods of helping individuals, families, groups and communities to meet their needs and to make the best use of the social services available.'[1] I should, however, want to make the qualification that (1) suggests more sociological knowledge than social workers can always claim. The question-begging term in this definition is of course 'needs'. In some branches of social work undoubtedly considerable attention is given to learning to diagnose what these are. But some of these needs may include the need to cope better morally with one's problems. The statement of the purpose of social work in the Younghusband Report is put in commendably simple language: 'The purpose of social work is to help individuals or families with various problems, and to overcome or lessen these so that they may achieve a better personal, family or social adjustment.'[2] This avoids being grandiose, but contains the question-begging term 'adjustment'. How much does 'adjustment' sometimes mean? A recent cartoon in *The New Yorker* has a lady consulting a psychiatrist who remarks: 'In a nutshell, Mrs Turner, either your son is making a remarkably fine adjustment to his lack of ability, or else he just doesn't care a damn.'

Because of the difficulty of defining an end which is partly at least a moral one, definitions of the purpose of social work tend, then, either to be put in very vague and rather grandiose language; or else the end is made to sound like a routine job of supplying practical help and

---

[1] Association of Social Workers, *A Report on Registration and the Social Worker*, London, 1955.

[2] *Report of the Working Party on Social Workers in the Local Authority Health and Welfare Services*, Her Majesty's Stationery Office, London, 1957, p. 7.

information. These are in effect the alternatives as Lady Wootton sees them; her own predilection is for the latter, and she is accordingly dubious whether an avocation so considered qualifies for professional status.[1] Moreover, she thinks that it is possible to separate the practical from the moral aspects of advice which may be given to people; to be efficient and sympathetic in giving the former, and permissive and tolerant in refraining from the latter.

But are these the alternatives? Is it not also possible to acknowledge in a rather more tough-minded way that there is a moral element in these activities? To begin with, can one really believe that all people's ideas about ways of life are equally good, including those that involve neglecting children and not paying the rent? When a probation officer is reported as having said at the Oxford Conference on 'Morals and the Social Worker' in 1959[2] that 'the purpose of casework is to free the client from his emotional troubles so that his own moral values can assert themselves', how many probation officers can put their hands on their hearts and say that this is really all that they are trying to do? (I note that other participants in that discussion had their doubts about how far one can take this 'permissive' attitude.) Many of those in the compulsory charge of a probation officer (in this case at any rate it seems a bit odd to call them 'clients') are not clear or stable enough in their own moral values for us to hope that these will 'assert themselves'. Some of them may not have anything coherent enough to be called a 'moral attitude'; others may need help in reshaping their attitude into one more satisfactory to themselves and less of a menace to other people than the attitude they hold now.

I am, of course, considering only the kinds of social work which are concerned with people's conduct. There may well be some services (for example supplying braille books to the blind, and a great many services which just call for practical information and help) where this problem need not arise. Where it does arise, is part of the trouble that the alternative possibilities tend to be stated incompletely? They are given as (a) 'permissiveness' (keeping one's own moral values out of it, and letting people make their own decisions), or (b) as an authoritarian judgemental attitude, or (c) as 'manipulation' (i.e. not telling a person what is what, but trying to get him where we want him by means of which he is not aware). Manipulation is very properly repudiated; but it is difficult to avoid it, if we do not realize clearly ourselves how much our moral values enter into the methods and ends we are pursuing.

[1] Barbara Wootton, *op. cit.*, p. 291.
[2] Association of Social Workers, *Morals and the Social Worker*, London, 1960.

But are these the only alternatives, any more than 'tolerating non-conformity' and 'pressures to conformity' are exhaustive alternatives? To take the latter disjunction first; there are surely deviants and deviants. Professor Roger Wilson for example distinguishes:

(1) Unconformity which offends neither the law, nor the conscience, nor the convenience of others, e.g. oddities of dress or eating habits.

(2) Unconformity by persons with an articulate conscience, e.g. rocket-site passive resisters.

(3) Unconformity by persons who are assumed to know the price in punishment or social isolation and are willing to risk having to pay it, e.g. the motoring offender, the big criminal, the petty delinquent who persists in committing crimes for rational gain, those with an 'unsettled way of life'.

(4) Unconformity which offends the law, the conscience or the convenience of others, and for which there is no satisfying rational explanation.[1]

It is doubtful whether these last nonconformists have very clear moral standards to assert. They may indeed have an inchoate cluster of moral sentiments, and in some of these—generosity for instance—they may leave many of us standing. But they need help in seeing what moral judgements mean. And is the skeleton in our cupboard that, unlike our Victorian forbears, we are not so sure what they mean ourselves?

Part of our trouble is the prevalence of the idea that moral standards are personal, subjective and emotional, and so are not matters into which intelligence enters, and for which reasons, maybe good reasons, can be given and communicated to other people. Alternative views are controversial, among moral philosophers no less than others. I should myself approach the question of moral judgement in a way which I can here only indicate sketchily. First, it is clear that no society can function without generally accepted *mores*, if for no other reason than that there must be some generally fulfilled expectations of how people will behave if anyone is to be able to carry out any purpose effectively. Next, any moral system will probably contain a number of obligations which, as time goes on, may seem odd, and sooner or later the question can be asked about any one of them, '*Why* ought I to do this?' Then legitimatizing reasons may be produced, some of which may also seem odd; they may include all sorts of authorities, traditions, discussions of desirable and undesirable consequences to oneself and others, and

---

[1] Roger C. Wilson, 'Unconformity in the Affluent Society', *Sociological Review*, Vol. VIII, No. 1, 1960.

appeals to more basic principles. If people are prepared to reveal these reasons and look at them, they can be discussed; some may be abandoned, some modified, and some reinforced. Their acceptance or rejection can then be a responsible matter, guided by some general notion of what morals are for—for instance, satisfactory ways of living with other people (this too is controversial; we need not claim to have the one correct moral philosophy, but only a reasonably grounded one). Whatever maxims we hold about how we think other people should behave, a reasonable defence of them implies that we should be prepared to see that what is sauce for the goose is sauce for the gander, and apply them to ourselves.

Thus, this is one respect in which a moral point can be put to a person as a matter of reason. One may be dealing with people who in effect expect exceptions in their own favour, and yet want to take advantage of the fact that other members of the community do not behave as they intend to behave themselves. This is an exercise demanding a certain amount of intellectual effort, though it need not be carried on in the technicalities of moral philosophy, and I suspect that more people than is always realized can engage in it, and in fact enjoy it. It would do no harm for social workers themselves to do more of it during their own training. Even if the result is to drive us back on to some moral principles or values for which we can give no further reasons, there will be a difference between holding them in this way *after* a process of critical heart-searching and just asserting them dogmatically. At any rate we can learn both to see moral questions as problematic and open ended, which means that they can be thought about and discussed, and also see there are reasonable ways of going about this.

To reach this point will mean helping social nonconformists of type 4 (the muddled and feckless) to turn into type 2, those who have their own moral will and convictions, however bizarre. There may well be many people who will never get to this point; and they probably will in fact need moral guidance and moral support. I met somewhere in the literature of social work the remark that 'the client is treated to less than a human relation if we don't discuss his problem as a moral problem with him'. I think that is profoundly true, except that all problems need not be moral ones. But it means that social workers must have done their own thinking about what a moral problem is like; and they must hold strongly enough that morality is part and parcel of any normal human life to believe that others will need to see some of their problems as moral problems too. This does *not* mean that one forces one's solution on them; but it does mean being prepared to throw one's intellectual moral resources as well as one's sympathetic ones into the situation. It may also mean that the relationship becomes a more adult one.

One rule should surely be that pressure must not be brought to bear on a client to do anything which he actually believes to be wrong (though the consequences of not doing it may be explained to him). This is well put in the 'Draft for a Code for Social Workers':[1] 'Respect for freedom of choice does not imply acquiescence in what is not right. But if a change is desirable, it should not be forced upon the client; the first effort should be directed towards enabling him to make the change himself' [but what do you do if he won't?*] 'It does imply respect for a client's moral standards' [but what if he needs to be shown how to acquire some?*]. 'The aim of a social worker should be to support, not to undermine a client's own standards, and solutions at variance with these should not be recommended.' When the client has made his own decision, the social worker may be able to help him even where he personally does not approve; but in instances where the decision is to do something which the social worker definitely believes is *wrong*, then he must surely be able to tell the client that he personally cannot help him implement it. This seems to me well put by Biestek.[2] Father Biestek writes from the background of a firm Thomist position; but those with a different moral philosophy can well learn from his clear thinking, and particularly from his analysis of the notion of 'acceptance': taking another person as he is, however unpleasant or uncongenial (cf. 'affective neutrality'), establishing a relation with him as he is, and refraining from passing judgement on his innocence or guilt, which does not mean necessarily approving of his behaviour and not wishing to help him change it. The general principle is that people should be helped to build up their own moral wills and their own integrity. And there may well be stages where they are so far from acting morally and responsibly (some children, for instance, delinquents, mentally sick people, and all of us at times, when for instance we need to be made to do something properly) that pressures of an educative kind are justified, so long as their purpose is to help us to become more capable of making responsible decisions in the end. There is a razor-edge balance needed here, for sometimes pressures may break down a person's own integrity; sometimes they may be the means

---

* Queries mine.
[1] *The Almoner*, 'Draft for a Code for Social Workers', Vol. III, No. 7, London, 1950.
[2] F. P. Biestek, *The Casework Relationship*, George Allen and Unwin, London, 1961.

of bringing him to the stage of being prepared to build it up. I am sure that a great deal more thinking needs to be done about the different kinds and uses of pressures. It will not be done if we assume that all pressure, and even indeed the moral influence of one person on another whom he is trying to help, must be eschewed.

I come back to the alleged invidiousness of the notion of 'doing good'. Perhaps what has brought it into disrepute is the suggestion that there are two kinds of people: the superior ones who can do good, and those who need to have good done to them. This can be broken down only if those who find themselves in positions where they are giving moral advice are also prepared sometimes to be at the receiving end. It is good that we should know people who knock us about morally, and that we should be able to get over the touchiness, insecurity, or self-esteem which makes us unwilling to expose ourselves to this sort of criticism. If we are prepared to do this, we can not only break down this most invidious of class distinctions, but also have a chance of learning more about the process of making moral judgements. For this is a skill, acquired like other skills, largely through its exercise. In these days when few of us think that we can look up the answers to moral problems at the back of a book, we may get further if we are prepared to take the risk of developing our powers of making moral judgements, rather than sit back and let these powers atrophy because of our uncertainties.

I began by saying that social workers lived at the uncomfortable, but at the same time potentially creative point where social science and psychology meet and are brought to bear on practical problems. I have now claimed that moral philosophy in the sense at least of a considered view of moral judgement, also intersects this point. Social work can, I believe, supply a field laboratory for the combination of these different ways of thinking; and if social workers can show how at any rate some parts of these ways of thinking can be made relevant to practical problems, they may not only help themselves by their exertions, but also help moral philosophers and social scientists by their example. But the job needs the co-operation of all these kinds of animal. Such co-operation might even do some good, in one of the less invidious senses of that expression.

2

PRINCIPLES AND ASSUMPTIONS UNDERLYING CASEWORK PRACTICE*

FLORENCE HOLLIS

Two groups of questions immediately come to mind which lead to the heart of our subject. First—what do we mean by the concept of acceptance? Shouldn't we let people know when we think they are doing the wrong thing? Doesn't one have to maintain one's own ethical standards? Isn't it insincere to pretend to agree when one does not? Second—what about this idea of self-determination? Don't we often know what is best for the client, what he ought to do and why then shouldn't we tell him what to do?

These at least set us on the way of re-examining our major assumptions. What *do* we mean by acceptance, and why have we come to believe in it? First of all, it is necessary to understand that acceptance refers to the feeling one has towards another. In essence it is a feeling of warmth, of positive good will, of a wish for the well-being of another person. We know that it is easy to have such feelings towards another who is likeable, who appeals to us, who is friendly to us, who behaves in a way that we can easily understand, towards which we naturally feel sympathetic. But our clients no more than other people are consistently like that. There are those who always see themselves in a favourable light, always mistreated, never at fault. There are those who mistreat their children, are actually cruel to them. There are those who impulsively throw over their responsibilities, or leave the convalescent home in an angry mood because they dislike the food after we have moved heaven and earth to get them in. Or is it just in the United States that we have these difficult people? Now we are not saying that one comes to *like* any of these ways of behaving, nor even that a caseworker never has feelings of irritation, even anger, at some of the ways of her clients. But what we are saying is that in order to help another person through

---

* A paper given at a United Nations seminar, Leicester, England, 1954.

the casework method there must be sufficient understanding of the need to act in this way, of the suffering that either precedes and causes, or else flows from such behaviour, to overshadow whatever feelings of irritation we experience and subordinate them to warm feelings of positive good will. Unless this atmosphere exists we have little indeed to offer our clients.

This attitude of acceptance of another person is quite different from approval of his behaviour. There are many times when we think our client is in the wrong, that his behaviour is unwise, to put it even more strongly, sometimes that his behaviour is truly wicked. Very frequently indeed, it is just because we think his behaviour is unwise that we should like to be able to help him to modify it through casework.

Nor does the attitude of acceptance necessitate any giving up of one's own personal code of ethics. It is not by any means a denial of values in behaviour. A sense of values the caseworker must have. Rather, it is a separation of judgements about values from feelings towards a person. Father Swithun Bowers in a recent article in *Social Casework*[1] makes a very good point in relation to this. He refers to the fact that we Americans have used the term 'non-judgemental' to describe this aspect of acceptance. He suggests that it would be more accurate to use the term 'non-condemnatory'. He is quite right in this, for the worker always has an opinion, a judgement, about his client's behaviour, but what he must not allow himself to do is to have feelings of condemnation towards his client because in his judgement the client is in the wrong. This is really a translation into casework terms of the age-old religious admonition to 'hate the sin but love the fellow sinner'. Indeed, it is only as the caseworker is able to feel the client's problem as a common human problem that is or very easily could be his too that true acceptance is possible.

As to the question of insincerity. Of course it would be insincere to pretend to agree or to approve when in truth we do not. There is nothing more important than honesty in the relationship between worker and client. But one does not have constantly to express agreement or approval to a client in order to demonstrate acceptance. Very frequently no expression of our opinion is called for at all, the important thing being for the client to arrive at his own thinking rather than to be told ours. At other times, it is quite possible effectively to raise questions about the advisability of a course the client is pursuing within the framework of an accepting relationship. Indeed, it is in this

[1] Swithun Bowers, O.M.I., 'Social Work and Human Problems', *Social Casework*, May, 1954, p. 187.

very atmosphere that our questions have the best chance of moving him to a re-examination of his own thinking. When we say then that casework is based upon a feeling of acceptance of the worker for the client, we mean that the worker feels warmth and good will and a wish for the client's well-being without feelings of condemnation towards him, whether his way of living pleases the worker or not.

What about self-determination, the second principle that raises so many perplexing issues? The word itself is misleading. It carries an emphasis on self and on independence which is sometimes interpreted to mean the right of the individual to pursue his own ends single-mindedly and with ruthless disregard for the rights or well-being of others. Nothing could be farther from the true meaning of the concept. Self-responsibility might even be a better term, for we are trying to describe the client's primary responsibility for the conduct of his own affairs. Wisely used, this includes his consideration of the rights and needs of others. But if he is to use this right wisely, he must have the opportunity to exercise it. The caseworker must not try to control his behaviour or make his decisions for him. This principle assumes that men do have a measure of choice in conduct of their own affairs, that behaviour is not mechanistically controlled and responsive in an automatic way to stimuli from the environment. It also assumes that this freedom to choose is translated into effective and satisfying choice in varying degrees by different people and that the more effectively the individual uses this latent power the more his own good and that of others is promoted. In order to use this power well, man must develop knowledge of himself and his work and must develop the power of control. These things come only as the result of the actual exercise of his freedom of choice. Therefore, we believe that the caseworker should promote rather than hinder the exercise of this power, and indeed that only in extreme situations should it be interfered with.

In actual practice, this is a very troublesome principle. Social work in my country has fully understood its implications only within the last twenty-five years. It is a principle too that is sometimes still honoured in the breach rather than in the observance. There are few things harder to do than to restrain oneself from subtly dominating other people, particularly so when it seems so obvious to us that we could lead their lives so much better than they can themselves! The caseworker's first question about this principle almost inevitably is—don't people have to be stopped from doing anti-social things? And of course the answer to this question is that in extreme instances they do have to be controlled. The right to self-direction is never an absolute.

At times we must take a protective role. A patient may be too sick mentally or physically to take responsibility for himself, or his behaviour may be so harmful to himself or to others that measures must be taken to restrain him. With children obviously this principle is subject to limitation because, in many respects, the child has neither the knowledge nor the maturity necessary for the complete conduct of his own affairs.

This then becomes a matter of judgement. We must decide when the principle of self-determination is superseded by the necessity for protection or direction. Here lies a great pitfall. It is a temptation to decide too readily that protective care is needed. The criteria can be so stretched as to make a farce of the principle. The burden of proof, it seems to me, lies upon the worker to demonstrate that protective or directive care is necessary. It should be resorted to only when other approaches have been tried without success and the situation is so serious that a change must take place. Even in the extreme example of a seriously psychotic patient, it is often possible, as we know, for the patient to take responsibility for his own voluntary commitment to a hospital. This in itself creates a more favourable atmosphere for psychiatric treatment. Furthermore, the fact that it is best for us to take responsibility for one facet of a person's life does not mean that his entire life need be under our supervision. If, in a parole situation, we of necessity control certain aspects of the parolee's life—we must exclude certain neighbourhoods as places to live, certain occupations, we must enforce certain regulations about his companions, his recreation, and so on—even within such strict limits as these, there are areas of life that need not be controlled by the parole officer, there are areas that can be made free for choice even within such regulations. The more these are used by the worker, the more the officer confines himself to the limitations that are unavoidable, the greater is his success with the parolee likely to be. I do not mean by this a weak or placating attitude where authority is necessary, but rather sufficient internal strength on the part of the worker to free him from the need to use authority unnecessarily.

Our next question about the client's right to conduct his own affairs really goes to the heart of the matter. Do we not in reality often know what is best for the client, and why then should we not tell him what to do? In the first place, it happens less frequently than we sometimes suppose that we do know what is best for the client. Usually our surest way to find out what is best for another person is to listen to his thoughts as we encourage him to explore the question for himself. Perceptive questions and comments, turning his attention to aspects of his problem which may have escaped him, are useful. But, by the time he has really expressed his own thoughts and feelings fully enough for us to have a worthwhile opinion about what it is wise for him to do, he has equipped himself with this same knowledge. He may not yet be ready to accept his own conclusions, but then neither would he be ready to follow our advice. Rather, the obstacles to his willingness to acknowledge what he knows becomes the next question to be explored. He will be far readier, however, to look at inconsistencies in his response to his own ideas than at his reluctance to accept ours. This is not to say that a caseworker never gives advice. There are times when we have knowledge of a situation that is beyond the client's knowledge. This is particularly true in health matters, often in educational and vocational matters, sometimes in aspects of child training. There are times when direct suggestions and direct advice about these things are very much in order, but advice that is given in an atmosphere of freedom for the client to reject the advice is quite different from that same advice given with the expressed or implied condition that the client is under obligation to accept and act upon it.

Why do we put all this stress upon self-direction? Because we believe it is one of the greatest dynamics of the whole casework approach. Because we believe that the soundest growth comes from within. Because we want to release the individual's own life energy to take hold of his situation. Because we believe there is within man a capacity for grasping the realities once he comes to understand them. Because we believe he is more satisfied with conclusions he arrives at through his own thinking even when those conclusions are painful ones. Because we believe that the more he exercises his innate capacity for decision making, for learning to see reality, the more that capacity will grow and the more he will be able to exercise it in his life after his association with the caseworker has ended. Because we have seen that somehow in this process energy is released, fears and timidities are reduced, self-confidence and self-respect grow, and people become better able to grapple with the frustrations and perplexities of their lives. But for this growth from within to occur there must be freedom— freedom to think, freedom to choose, freedom from condemnation, freedom from coercion, freedom to make mistakes as well as to act wisely. Strength to understand and to act upon one's understanding comes only as one actually experiences and exercises the freedom to direct one's own thoughts and behaviour—and that is what we mean by self-determination in casework practice.

Here another knotty question rears its head. Is there not an inconsistency in our believing so firmly in the acceptance of the client and in his right to self-direction on the one hand, and our having in our own minds on the other hand treatment goals towards which we are trying to move him, although he may not himself even know what these goals are? For instance, a wife comes in complaining of her husband's lack of interest and of his criticism of her for over-eating which has caused her to become unattractively fat. When she first comes in it is in a complaining mood. Consciously or unconsciously she wants our sympathy and wants us to change her husband's behaviour toward her. We, on our side, immediately begin in our minds to wonder whether she on her part is doing something to provoke her husband's lack of interest, and we wonder why she is over-eating. At first we listen receptively, seeking to understand, but soon we begin to form the opinion that our client is over-reacting to a certain degree of irritating domination by her husband, that she is bringing his criticism down on her head by reacting negatively to both reasonable and unreasonable requests, and that her over-eating is in part a negative displaced reaction from her childhood when her mother nagged her about over-eating, and in part a deliberate though unconscious effort to displease her husband. Immediately a potential treatment goal begins to form itself in our mind. Could she be helped to see that she over-reacts to her husband, that she purposely irritates him, that she reacts to him irrationally as to her mother? Further than that, can she be helped to understand why she does these things, can she actually work through some of her early feeling about her mother so that she will not be merely controlling her hostile response but will be rid of the need for it? The answer to questions such as these rests upon many things— upon our estimate of the degree of health or illness in the client's total personality, upon the worker's degree of training and skill, upon the nature of the agency to which the client comes, but ultimately it rests upon two other things of over-riding importance—upon the client's willingness to seek this understanding, and upon the value system within which the caseworker practices.

It is absolutely impossible to make a person develop understanding about himself against his will. It is only if our treatment goals are clearly subordinated in our own minds to this condition that we will have a favourable atmosphere for these goals also to become the client's. In other words, the help we offer is the product of our general knowledge of personality and social conditions, of our understanding of this individual and his situation, and of our value system. The help the client uses must be consistent with his own vision for himself. If this wife never moves beyond the desire for sympathetic understanding and modification of her husband we will be able to help her only on this level. As a matter of fact, during the first few months of treatment with her first worker this was exactly what did happen.

The wife's bitterness towards her husband was reduced considerably by her pouring out to the caseworker her feeling about his demands upon her and his lack of warmth towards her. The husband also came in for interviews, in the same fashion expressed his feeling and, to a certain extent, recognized the irritating effect on his wife of some of his behaviour. As a result of these things there was some improvement in their relationship to each other. Then because the first worker left the agency a new caseworker began interviews with the couple.

The second worker offered more and the client used more. It was part of the second worker's task to help the client to overcome her resentment and fear of criticism enough to allow herself to look at her own part in her own troubled life and to accept for herself the goal of greater self-understanding and control. Ultimately the wife was able to do this. She gained understanding of her own over-reaction to her husband and of the ways in which she herself stimulated him to the very behaviour of which she complained. Further, she was then able to modify her responses to him so that a substantial change in their whole relationship took place.

At the outset it was in this situation, as it is in every other, an open question as to whether or not the client could accept and participate in this kind of help. To succeed the worker had to be ready on her part to accept the client's decision and to help on the level the client chose. In other words, a dual responsibility is involved for the worker. He must offer the highest level of assistance which he is equipped to give and which he believes the client may be able to use, and must exercise his highest skill in overcoming the client's resistance to using this degree of help, but at the same time he must refrain from coercive methods and must at all times be willing to offer help of a more limited type if this is what the client ultimately wants and can use. Only under these conditions is there compatibility between our acceptance of the client and of his right to self-direction and our formulation of treatment goals towards which we hope to motivate him.

What of the value system within which the caseworker operates? We have said that the principle of acceptance does not in any way imply that the caseworker is without a value system of his own. This will vary with different individuals and will inevitably condition what the caseworker offers the client. Caseworkers are not all alike. We each have our characteristic ways of working, and this includes the way in which our work is affected by our own goals and ideals. Over and above this, however, I believe we can agree on certain values which are characteristic of casework itself—or perhaps of social work itself. These are certainly among the principles and assumptions which underly case-practice. Perhaps this is a good place to comment on my general orientation to this afternoon's subject. Here, as elsewhere in this paper, I am inevitably influenced by casework as I know it and practice it. I am not trying to define principles that would necessarily be accepted by social work the world over.

Some of the principles of casework practice rest upon scientific findings, others upon the accumulated experience and intuitions of our social and religious culture. Indeed, one of the most interesting things about these values is the extent to which scientific findings so often converge with principles previously established through social and religious experience. An excellent example of this is our present assumption about the relationship between love, hate and fear. Religion has long taught that the chief evil in the world is hate, the desire to hurt another, and that fear is an outcome of hate, that hate must be overcome by love, and that when this occurs fear will be cast out, will disappear. The findings of analytic psychology are that the individual struggles between the creative love instinct and the destructive death instinct, that the love instinct must somehow come to bind the death instinct if love rather than hate is to predominate in the individual's life, and that anxiety—fear—of various types springs ultimately from the individual's inability to subordinate his wish to harm to his wish to love. This to me is the basic premise upon which casework rests. Our conception of the casework relationship is essentially that the worker's good will towards the client is a necessary component to his improvement —good will, acceptance—these are forms of love. Our major goals in treatment are to increase the individual's ability to love, either to decrease his hate and hostility, or to enable him better to control his hate and hostility, and to convert destructive aggression into constructive and even creative aggression. We do this in many ways— sometimes by reducing the frustration of the environment, sometimes by the giving of reassurance and appreciation which decreases the individual's feeling of being unloved or unlovable and hence hostile, sometimes by trying to drain off some of the angry feelings in harmless or less harmful directions. At other times we use the healing power of the accepting relationship itself, we help the person to understand the causes of his underlying hostility and thus be rid of them, or we offer creative outlets for aggression through which destructive anger can find a constructive use. There are many casework tools and methods but all are used in accordance with the underlying assumption that love must be strengthened and hostility or hate somehow bound, and that through this anxiety and fear will be lessened and energy for more satisfying living will be released.

A related assumption upon which casework operates is that the individual is happier, has greater satisfaction in life, in proportion to the extent to which his capacity to love others has outgrown his love of himself. This is a curious concept and always hard to state because in actuality the person who is truly able to love others also loves himself. It is only when the latter exists without the former, or with very little of the former, that the individual's life is narrowed, warped and embittered. Here again we see a convergence of scientific findings and religious and social experience. In analytic terms incorporated into casework thinking we speak of the development from narcissism to object love. And by object love we mean the capacity to see people as they are in reality rather than as we want them to be in our fantasy, and to love them for what they are, to want to contribute to their happiness, rather than to love them only for being what we want them to be and for their contribution to our happiness. This underlying assumption is converted into practice whenever it is possible to do so by helping one person better to understand another—the husband his wife, the mother her child, the child his parents. Indirectly many of the same processes are used as in the struggle between love and hate, for for more mature love is often unable to develop because the energy is bound in old hostilities and feelings of bitterness. If you doubt the validity of my saying that these two assumptions underly casework practice, let me ask you—have you ever made it your ultimate treatment goal to increase either hostility or self-centredness? You may often have sponsored the expression of hostility, but that was either for the purpose of ultimately reducing it or as a step in channelling it into constructive activity in changing a damaging life situation in which the client was caught. Again, the ultimate purpose was that of reducing unnecessary suffering and hence the response of destructive aggression. You may have encouraged more self-assertiveness and self-gratification, but was not that when your client had in reality turned hostility against himself, depriving himself because of his fear of his unrecognized and unresolved anger at others? The underlying assumption upon which you operate is that ultimately there will be less hostility and the capacity for more object love.

A third principle to which I believe casework adheres is that men are more likely to act wisely in the best interests of others and of themselves when they understand themselves and others. In other words, that action based on knowledge is superior to blind obedience. With this in mind, we seek constantly to broaden and deepen our client's understanding of their situations, of other people, of their own feelings and reactions. This is a slower method for immediate results than that of giving active direction, but it is our assumption that in the long run the client will act more wisely and will achieve more lasting ability to manage his affairs as his ability to understand them grows. We know that sometimes clients are not able to use this approach and of course there are many aspects of casework in which the problem is not one of lack of understanding, but where it is, and the client can respond on this level, it is our belief that he will achieve the greatest measure of improvement if he can gain greater knowledge of his situation, his associates, and himself.

But why do we care about these things? Why do we go to all this trouble? Why do we have such a thing as social work anyway? Are there not some even more fundamental assumptions than these that underly our casework practice? Yes, I think there are. Fundamental to all else is the belief that human life is precious, that the individual has the right to grow and develop and achieve the highest degree of happiness or satisfaction in life of which he is capable. This in turn, we believe, depends upon his functioning at the height of his own capacities—intellectual, physical, emotional and spiritual capacities. We believe, too, that there are inter-relationships between the well-being of one person and that of another—that man cannot live well for himself alone. The lives of individuals are so enmeshed that one person can only be helped as he is seen in relation to the others with whom he is closely associated. He can only steer his own course successfully as he considers it in relation to others. Indeed the very existence of social work itself is an expression of this belief. It rests upon the idea that one individual has responsibility for enhancing the welfare of another. Collectively through social institutions we carry out this responsibility. Otherwise we would believe in the survival of the fittest and would not waste our time looking after those who have run behind in the race. But we are slowly coming to realize that there is no sharp line between the fit and the unfit, that the concept of the survival of the fittest applied to human lives results ultimately in destruction for all.

We also believe that in their essential value as human beings all men are equal. This has many implications. Social work does not discriminate between races, or nationalities, between rich and poor, between educated and uneducated in the quality of service it gives. Even though in the lives of our countries—and I speak for my own—this ideal has been very imperfectly achieved, social work itself can be found in the vanguard of those who seek to break down the inequalities between men and to offer opportunities and services which will in some measure compensate for their deprivations.

Related to this is also our belief in the value of diversity. Social work does not strive for uniformity. Rather, we believe that many patterns of life are possible and useful and that each individual will fashion his own particular solution to his problems and find a mode of life that establishes his own equilibrium. In fact we welcome this diversity because we believe it enriches life for all of us as well as giving greater play to each person's creativity. Hence in our work we seek to free the individual to find his own way of life, not to imitate ours. In our supervision we encourage the student to keep his own spontaneous and natural way of relating to people, of expressing himself, rather than to imitate the style of his teachers. A certain amount of imitating he will of course do, but this we regard as a stage of transition which he may need to lean on until he can establish his own characteristic ways of working. It is for this reason that we tend to discourage observation of interviews of more experienced workers. This assumption applies also to diversity in the practice of casework in different countries. It would be a very great mistake to think that either training or practice can be identical in different countries. Individual variations there must be. We can assimilate only so much from each other. We must integrate what we learn from each other into the peculiar fabric of our own culture and situations, never slavishly copy. The strange part of it is that the freer we are to do this the more we are likely in reality to learn and, in turn, to contribute.

An assumption that is sometimes overlooked, especially by younger caseworkers, is that there is value in the relief of suffering itself. The student in particular is so often interested only in cure—in helping the person to change, to function on a higher level, to be rid of his handicap. This has certain advantages for sometimes the very aspiration of the young worker makes the impossible possible. But no one can be content in social work or truly effective in social work if he sets his goal always at positive change. There are so many times that all we can do is to alleviate suffering, to help the person bear his misfortunes. That this in itself is worth doing is one of the fundamental premises upon which casework is based.

These, then, are some of the components of the value system within which the caseworker operates. The help he offers inevitably falls within this framework. The goals towards which he hopes the client will move must be consistent with it. The framework is broad enough to permit many different kinds and levels of help suited to the needs and wishes of a wide variety of people. Whether or not the client wants this help and how much of what is offered he wants to use remains his own decision.

There is another set of assumptions or principles upon which casework rests—assumptions that have to do not with values and goals but with the relationship of casework to scientific method. Casework originally was based largely on intuition and common sense. These two ingredients are certainly indispensable to modern practice though some of our critics accuse us of having done away with them long since. To them we have added the use of scientific method. This means that we now give allegiance to certain scientific assumptions. The first of these is that human behaviour is governed by psychological and social laws rather than being erratic and accidental. Once this premise is accepted it opens the door to the study of causation in behaviour. This, in turn, leads to the assumption that when behaviour is understood it becomes susceptible to change by consciously directed processes. It is further assumed that it is possible for the laws of human behaviour to be discovered and understood with constantly improving fullness and exactness through such scientific methods of study as observation, comparison, inference, hypothesizing, classifying, generalizing, and testing or validating. This means that workers must be trained in accurate observation and recording, must be familiar with what is already reasonably well established about human behaviour and must in their work think of the individual they are trying to help in relation to this body of knowledge.

The gradual incorporation of scientific method into casework practice has raised many questions for us. I should like again to use the approach of discussing issues as they are typically raised, sometimes by beginners and sometimes by seasoned workers in our field.

The first question to be raised about these scientific principles is often the philosophical one of whether the assumption of lawfulness in behaviour and of cause and effect relationships in behaviour does not mean that casework has become completely deterministic. How can this be reconciled with the principle of self-determination as we discussed it earlier in this paper? As you know, this is a problem with which philosophers have struggled these many centuries. The case-

c

work position, I would think, would not be that of absolutism in either direction. We certainly do not take the libertarian stand that each action of man is completely free and unaffected by his previous charac-- ter, life history or current experience. On the other hand, neither do we believe that all choice, all behaviour is the determined, necessary and inflexible result of previously existing physical or environmental causes. Rather, we believe that there exists a measure of freedom influenced by constitutional factors, previous life experiences and the current environment. Through scientific method we hope to under- stand these latter factors and hence to modify them, or to use them in the pursuit of individual and social goals. The concept of lawfulness excludes the possibility of freedom and spontaneity in behaviour only when lawfulness is considered synonomous with exact repetition and frequency.

A similar question, again of a philosophic nature, is that of whether casework is committed to positivism, the doctrine that knowledge must be based exclusively on the methods and discoveries of science. This is not a necessary corollary of the adoption of scientific method as long as we do not arbitrarily exclude certain areas of life from scientific study. To use scientific methods to learn what can be learned by those methods does not necessarily commit one to the belief that this is the only source of knowledge. As to whether or not there are other kinds of knowledge, different workers will have different opinions. The adoption of scientific methods to study and to understand as much as can be known by these methods is all that modern casework asks of its practitioners. It will be a long time before we approach the ultimate limits of that knowledge.

A particularly difficult stumbling block for many workers and students has to do with the scientific process of classification or, as it is sometimes critically called, categorization. Are we not, the argument runs, destroying individuality, denying the uniqueness of the indivi- dual and distorting reality when we place a person in a category? If we truly placed a whole person in a category, this would certainly be a valid criticism. But if we do this, we are misusing the concept of classification. We are confusing the part with the whole. One does not properly classify people. One classifies the behaviour or the situation of people. When we say, for instance, that a given man is a compulsive neurotic, what we really mean is that he behaves to a marked degree in a compulsively neurotic way in certain respects—that he behaves in a fashion similar to other people suffering from a similar personality disturbance—disturbance of behaviour. Or when we say that this child is an orphan, we really mean that he has been orphaned—that he is in an orphaned situation—his parents have died. It is when we are confused on this point that we run into stereotyping. Stereotyping or categorizing occurs when we form in our minds a composite picture of a given classification and confuse that composite picture with the live person whose behaviour places him in that classification. Then in truth we do injustice to that individual—and we will do poor casework as well.

All people are both unique and like others in their behaviour—in their feelings, in their thoughts, in their actions. We must not lose sight of either of these characteristics. We must be well attuned to the individual variations, the unique flavour, the essence that characterizes the alive human being with whom we are working, and our treatment methods are never absolutely the same for any two people. It would be an impossibility. At the same time, we must recognize that there is also a great deal of similarity in the behaviour of human beings and that some people are more alike than others. People fall into sub-groupings of closer resemblance in their behaviour when they either are similar in constitutional make-up, or have had similar developmental experiences, or meet similar life experiences. It is because this is true that we can understand each other and that we can build up a body of accumulated knowledge which enables us to understand and help more quickly, because we bring to the new person who comes to us all that we know about helping other people who have had similar experiences and have reacted in similar ways.

The correct use of classification also depends upon the nature of the classification itself and upon our own understanding of the meaning of the classification. The more a classification merely puts together the superficial outward manifestations of behaviour, the less useful it will be. The more it succeeds in putting together behaviour that springs from similar causative factors and similar dynamics, the more useful it will be.[1] Furthermore, our knowledge of any classification we use must be so complete that we keep in mind not just descriptively what it means but also dynamically and genetically what it means—the life experiences that have probably contributed to it, the feelings experienced by the person who typically reacts in a given way.

For instance, in thinking of a compulsive person we must think of the strict demands for conformity that his parents must have placed upon him, of his wish to please them, combined with his resentment at

---

[1] See Kurt Lewin's 'The Conflict between Aristotelian and Galileian Modes of Thought in Contemporary Psychology', in the *Journal of General Psychology*, 1931, pp. 141–177, for a full discussion of this and related subjects.

having to please them. We must think of how he has now made these demands his own and of how he fears not to live up to them and drives himself and others to live up to them, of how he is trying so hard to keep his anger about it all inside, letting it out only when he thinks he can justify it, and of how he has to develop all kinds of rigidities to control his feelings, and of how guilty he feels when they become too strong and overwhelm him, and of how he so often has to reassure himself by a façade of self-righteousness and the ultimate of correctness in behaviour. And further, we must understand his underlying fear and his discomfort in all this and how hard he is trying to do what he thinks is right and how afraid he is that what he does is not right and that no one will love him. If we can bring all that to bear upon our approach to a compulsive person, will we not in our effort to understand and help him be many steps ahead of where we would be if we had to wait until we understood his whole individual life history before piecing together his strange and often unpleasant behaviour?

One further warning about classification. In actuality, behaviour is a continuum. In the strict sense of the word, no arbitrary boundary can be set up between two closely related classifications, each merges into the next. This is the most clearly seen in the use of the Intelligence Quotient. Individuals whose intelligence quotient falls between 50 and 74 are commonly known as morons or dullards. Those below 50 are called imbeciles, and those above 74 are considered normal. Now certainly the moron with an IQ of 74 and a normal person with an IQ of 75 are more alike than the moron of 74 and the moron of 50. Classification is a convenience for breaking down our total knowledge into manageable units, but classification must be used with full recognition of its relationship to the continuous nature of differences between people and with full awareness of the individuality of the specific person and degree to which his behaviour falls within a category.

It sometimes happens that we become afraid of so much 'science' in casework. Quite rightly we fear its becoming routinized, a matter of following rules, a matter of book-learning.

Is there then in modern casework no place for intuition, we ask? What is intuition? It is the direct apprehension of a reality. It is a form of insight. Strictly speaking, intuition is always accurate. If it is false, it is only a pseudo-intuition—a delusion, a bias taken as truth. The capacity for intuition is the most valuable natural quality the caseworker can possess. In his day-by-day work it enables him correctly and directly to perceive what his client is feeling and perhaps something of the cause and solution of his problem. In the building of a body of knowledge about people and how to help them, intuition is the primary means by which new insights are gained. How many times in the history of science all the facts on which a new formulation was based have been known and before the eyes of all to see. It was their significance that escaped the view of all until someone intuitively sensed their meaning and propounded a theory to embrace the facts. Sometimes the intuition, the hunch, comes first before the facts are marshalled, and the facts have to be painstakingly sought to test the hunch to see whether it was truly intuition or merely a plausible idea.

The problem then becomes one of how does one develop intuition and how does one distinguish between true and false intuitions and avoid the latter. I doubt if we can altogether avoid having pseudo-intuitions. When the mind is free to react spontaneously, errors are bound to occur. But we can always check our hunches before we act upon them and this applies whether it is a sudden insight into what a client is saying in an interview or a new concept about behaviour or treatment that can be tested either in experimentation or against the findings of others.

Can the capacity for true intuition be developed? I think it can and that it is cultivated by the very things that we strive for in the caseworker's relationship with his client. That is not to say that everyone has the same talent for intuition. We know that there are great individual variations in this but, nevertheless, what talent there is can either be developed or stunted in its growth. We seek in the casework relationship, do we not, to feel into—einfuhlen—the other person; to have empathy for him. This calls for a quality of loving attention. You have to care enough about finding out, care enough about helping to invest your libido exclusively in this person for this moment. The product of these flashes of insight, combined with the other things we know about this person and his situation and with our general theoretical knowledge, enables us to help him. There are two hazards in this process against which we try to build protections. One is that we will become lost in our empathy with the client, that we will become so identified with him that we are as enmeshed and helpless in his problem as he is himself. Empathy alone is not enough. It must be in the service of the worker's independent judgement. On the other hand, empathy must not be confused with projection into the client of the worker's thoughts and reactions. That is the very opposite of empathy and is a product really of self-absorption on the part of the worker instead of absorption in the person needing our help. This does not mean that the worker is without reactions to the client. On the contrary, our own reactions, if we are aware of them, can become another source of knowledge about the client. These, after all, are one index of how his behaviour affects other people and can be used in understanding if we can recognize them for what they are. Thus, they, too, can feed into both our intuitive and our learned understanding of our client. No, we assuredly do not find incompatibility between the use of intuition in casework practice and its reliance on scientific method.

We have ranged over many assumptions today. There are others. Each of us faced with this assignment would find himself impelled to a somewhat different selection—thus exercising our spontaneity and freedom of choice—but on the whole I suspect we would find that in one way or another we stressed many of these same principles. We begin with acceptance, the dispassionate commitments to the well-being of the person we are trying to help. We make positive use of the individual's capacity for self-direction by jealously guarding his freedom of choice. We are guided in the help we offer by our value assumptions that man and his fulfillment are intrinsically valuable, that men are mutually dependent and bear responsibility for each other, that men are equal in their essential value and rights, that man's destructive tendencies must be held in leash and overbalanced by the strength of his love, as he moves in the direction of love turned outward rather than inward. We use in our work the scientific method with its assumptions that there is lawfulness in human affairs and that painstaking study, illuminated by intuition, can bring us a progressively clearer appreciation of truth.

3

THE SOCIAL WORKER AND HIS SOCIETY*

GRACE LONGWELL COYLE

ONE of the characteristics of any profession is that it has a specific function not only defined by its practitioners but recognized and sanctioned by its society. As those familiar with the history of social work know, defining our function has not been simple. We seem now to have arrived at one stage which, even if it does not provide us with a slogan that can make us popular with public relations experts, at least gives us a clearer direction for our own efforts.

We are increasingly used to the distinction between the social welfare services as such and the profession of social work which has developed within them. I shall not pause here to attempt exact definition of the type of services now commonly designated in such terms as 'the social services' or 'social welfare services'. These are, I think, well known. My main concern is focused rather on social work as the profession that has developed within the social welfare services for the purpose of making them as valuable as possible to their clientele and as effective as possible in fulfilment of the social goals that led society to establish them. The development of needed social welfare services and preparation for their effective administration should be the major concerns of the professional schools. Related to this is preparation for the practice of social work, to which I wish to direct chief attention. As the functions of the social services have multiplied and differentiated themselves, it has become clear that several kinds of knowledge, skill, and expertness are required for their effective administration. This knowledge and skill and the professional attitudes and ethics involved have developed over the last forty years into the functions of the present-day social worker.

Exactly what is the major characteristic of the service we call social work? As a basis for consideration, I should like to use a part of a definition recently developed by Harriett Bartlett: 'The central focus of

* Published in *The Social Service Review*, Vol. XXX, No. 4, December, 1956.

social work is upon the understanding of the social situation and its meaning to the individual or group . . . The term "psychosocial" is often used to describe this concern with the inner and outer factors (or with the interaction of physical, emotional, social, and cultural factors).'[1]

More concretely, this means, in the first place, those relations between person and person upon which much of the stability and enhancement of life depends and in which the deepest needs for mutual affection and respect find their satisfaction. These are the familiar substance of our daily practice—the child without parents, the family in conflict, the home disrupted by the mother's illness, the family wishing to adopt a child, the adolescent group of friends seeking more satisfying outlets for their energies, the old people without friends or companions, the group in a children's ward of a hospital.

In these situations the psychosocial elements are relations between person and person. There is also much of our practice in which the relation is between a person and his society. 'The party of the second part', as the lawyers would say, is not another person but a social situation. The man unemployed because of automation, the Mexican migrant family wintering in the city, the Negro white-collar worker unable to find suitable housing—these and many other situations present us with the psycho-social problems inherent in a constantly expanding economy, a mobile population, a society still characterized by social barriers and stratifications.

This substance of social work practice consists of an infinite variety of psychosocial factors—some between person and person, some between a person and his society. What is it we do with such situations? In some cases we are dealing with maladjustments or disfunctioning, as in the family in conflict or the migrant Mexicans unfamiliar with the demands of urban life. In some cases we are dealing with lacks—the emotionally disturbed adolescent unable to make friends among his peers, the old person whose friends and family are no longer there, the cardiac child separated from family and friends in a hospital ward, the child awaiting adoption. In still others we are dealing with the enrichment and enhancement of social relations necessary to growth, as, for example, in the provision for the close-knit friendship groups of adolescents and the group work services in a home for emotionally disturbed girls. Although these may seem outwardly different, they are in fact parts of a whole—assistance to people in creating, maintaining,

---

[1] Harriett M. Bartlett, 'Fifty Years of Social Work in the Medical Setting', (paper presented at the Massachusetts General Hospital, Boston, on October 22, 1955, at the fiftieth anniversary of the Social Service Department.

and enhancing those basic social relationships upon which the security and happiness of the individual depends.

As I have reflected upon this phrase, 'psychosocial adjustment', it has seemed to me that we are sometimes like a musician trying to play an intricate piece of music with hands that are not equally developed. With the 'psycho' hand we have, especially in recent years, developed especial skills based upon a well-founded theoretical base and adapted now to the special function of the social worker. The 'social' hand, it seems to me, is still at the level of finger exercises or playing intuitively by ear. The equivalent theory regarding society or culture is not as yet fully known or as appropriately applied. At times we seem to be almost tone deaf on that side. If I am focusing on the social aspects of social work, it is in the hope that we shall in time develop more fully our understanding of the social causes that underlie the problems with which we deal and, in some cases, the social measures required for their treatment. For the full rendering of the intricate score that confronts us as social workers, both hands must be used if we are to create that essential harmony of the individual and the social which is our ultimate goal.

If, then, this concern with psychosocial relations is its essential focus, what does social work contribute to society today, and how is it related to that society? I should like to present three propositions which seem in part the answers to these questions. In the first place, our society apparently produces, by the way it functions, a need for assistance in such psychosocial relations, and in many cases this need can be met only by the social welfare provisions, public and private, through which social work service is available. In the second place, social workers have a 'public health' function for the prevention of these social conditions or for their amelioration. Such a public health function requires not only services to individuals but changes in the social situation itself. Third, social work goal and values are themselves a significant contribution to our surrounding society.

Services to individuals.—Elton Mayo[1], writing ten years ago on the 'seamy side of industrial progress', was among the first to point out that our society, with its demand for flexibility, logical thinking, social mobility, and highly technical work skills, was producing an unusual crop of unhappy individuals and of conflicting groups. He warned us that, unless we found ways to develop equally effective social skills by which people learned to live in such a society, we were headed for

[1] Elton Mayo, *The Social Problems of an Industrial Civilization*, Graduate School of Business Administration, Harvard University, Boston, 1945, pp. 6-15.

social disaster. While the older, established societies taught the social skills of personal relationships and co-operative effort within the network of relatively stable family and community living, the new adaptive society has required major modification not only in work habits but in the basic social relations of life. The resulting social disruption creates drifting individuals who are without meaningful community roots and are incapable of deep stable personal ties.

In recent years the chorus of social comment to this effect has swelled from many sides. Psychiatrists warn us of the increase in character disorders among the young; sociologists describe the conforming masses of persons who have no ability to develop into free autonomous beings or to participate with independence in the creation of a democratic community life. Eric Fromm describes the threat to personality as that of schizoid alienation that turns men into robots easily subject to the manipulation of the all-powerful state.[1]

Perhaps this thesis, now familiar to most of us, is best summed up in some vivid phrases by Max Lerner. 'Latter day man', according to this theory, he says, 'within his new society is surrounded by automatism, battered by sounds and images hurled at him as a target, pressured toward conformity; he wanders lonely as an alienated cloud over a wilderness of commodities . . .'[2]

My own reaction to some of these prophecies of doom is to view them as somewhat exaggerated and oversimplified diagnoses of our social situation. The human animal is a very resilient creature, and if he cannot find nourishment for his social needs in the accustomed ways he is likely to invent new ones—often not visible because new to those who sit in a lofty isolation condemning him to alienation, conformity, and social dislocation. A closer look would reveal the enormously complex and meaningful network of personal relationships that penetrate all places of work and many neighbourhoods, the satisfactions which create and maintain our many vast voluntary organizations, churches, unions, political parties, or women's clubs. In saying this, I do not mean that these largely obscure but pervasive primary relations in work place and neighbourhood provide all the social nourishment required, nor that the impact of the large secondary groups is in fact satisfying in the same useful ways which were available in the stable community life of earlier times, though they may mitigate the social situation described. It seems obvious that there is something to be said

[1] Eric Fromm, 'The Present Human Condition', *American Scholar*, Vol. XXV, winter, 1955-6, 29-35.
[2] Max Lerner, 'The Flowering of Latter Day Man', *American Scholar*, Vol. XXV, winter, 1955-6, 27. (Mr Lerner does not entirely agree with this diagnosis.)

for this diagnosis of our society and, moreover, that in so far as it is true it is a major concern of the social work profession.

In fact, as one reflects on these criticisms of our society and the accompanying warnings of social doom, one is struck by the fact that perhaps these phenomena of social dislocation and disruption, of personal isolation and rootlessness, may be the very source out of which our profession among others has grown. Behind the rise and increase of the varieties of such professions there must be some widespread need for help in social relations. Psychiatrists, counselling services, and group therapies of many kinds, as well as the vast amount of advice to the lovelorn and the popular courses for improving one's personality, all bear witness to the fact that our society does produce a host of unhappy individuals seeking somehow the way out of lonely alienation or interpersonal conflict into a life in which the basic psychological need for affection, stability, and growth can be met in fruitful social relations. Social work is obviously not the only or even the largest of the occupations which have arisen in the last fifty years as the new society has borne its fruit of high productivity, and fabulous technological achievement, and, perhaps as a consequence, its crop of unhappy individuals and conflicting groups.

Social work, however, while not the largest or—we are told—the most highly rated among such occupations, is, I believe, one of the soundest. By this I mean it is attempting to develop its practice responsibly on the basis of the careful assimilation and use of the best scientific knowledge it can find and master. It is constantly attempting to analyse its methods. Its basic concern is without question the welfare of its clientele, and it has developed a responsible ethic which gives direction to its use of the knowledge it acquires. It has, in short, the characteristics of a profession, although a relatively young one with much yet to be done in its development.

Let us take a look, then, at what social work has learned and is doing which has bearing on this malady of our society. What can we claim today as our contribution to the psychosocial relations with which we deal? Where could we do more?

Obviously, in such a paper it would be not only impractical but presumptuous to try to give the answers to such questions. Perhaps, in fact, I can only provide more questions—often the beginning of wisdom. What I can present is obviously the evaluation by one person and no doubt one with a particular angle. As I see it, then, we can claim the following kinds of contribution to the problems outlined above.

Our first and perhaps most clearly recognized function lies in the preservation and enhancement of family relationships. It is the family—its present instability, its loss of function, its confusion as to its authority and the roles of its members—which creates the most concern among observers of our social scene. It is here that social work has put much of its effort and has concentrated its most highly skilled practice. It is here that the use of psychoanalytic theory has made its most appropriate and deepest impact.

At the present time two very significant changes are evident in our approach to the family. In the first place, the tendency to treat the family as such—as a group—rather than to focus on the individual, with only a peripheral vision of his family relations, is a move away from a completely individual and largely intrapsychic concern. Second, we seem to be moving also towards seeing each family in its cultural and social setting. There is wider realization, born from the recent marriage of anthropology and psychiatry, that the family is a social institution with differing distributions of roles and methods of child-rearing in various parts of our society. With this will come not only a more adequate understanding of individual behaviour as in part a cultural product transmitted through the family as its bearer. There will also be born a clearer recognition that the family is not one set of relations but many and that our approach to it must be related to the changing norms and social conditions of its cultural milieu. We are, in such developments, moving towards the deeper understanding of the 'social' term in psychosocial relations to match more expertly the more highly developed skills already acquired in the 'psycho' term of our function.

This skill and experience with the maintenance of families will remain and expand as one of our major contributions to social stability and individual fulfilment. What was discovered and started among the families of the poor is now available for use with necessary modifications in other parts of our society.

I should like also to review briefly what seem to me to be the major contributions of the group worker to the social ailment with which we started. If this seems perhaps overemphasized, you will no doubt lay it to my own bias.

The group worker, like the family caseworker, deals with primary-group relations, that is, with face-to-face relations primarily in small groups which involve the members in attachments and activities of considerable meaning. In thet hirty years since we first began to look intensively at such relations in social agencies we have come to understand increasingly the patterns of group interaction, group modes of behaviour, group pathologies and distortions, the opportunities group experience affords for the expansion of the self and for growth in social usefulness. We still have a long way to go, but some of our effort has already borne fruit in more sensitive understanding, more effective relations between worker and group, and, we believe, in greater human happiness and growth.

In discussing the breakdown of the old ways of training people in the social skills Elton Mayo has pointed out that what society does not provide naturally or without thought must be consciously and plan-fully invented. I have sometimes thought that this was the true origin of group work, though as usual its originators responded with only partial awareness to this new and as yet undefined social need. This is particularly evident in the provision under social agency auspices of the play group for the pre-adolescent, the social club of the early adolescent years, the courtship activities of middle adolescence and young adult-hood. The spirit of youth in the city streets often found itself frustrated and bored because of lack of outlets, or involved in antisocial or at best futile enterprises, many of which were outside the direction of the family or of an actively functioning neighbourhood control. More by insight than by knowledge, the answer evolved in the clubs, classes, and other activities, and, later, as we began to see more what we were really doing, in the attempt to understand and to use the spontaneous demands of youth for meaningful social relations as the means for richer development along socially useful lines.

As we have worked at this we have evolved certain experiences which could and should be more widely used. One is a realization of the essential part that such group experience plays in the maturing process of the growing child and youth. The need to function outside the parental family, to make his way with his own generation, to give and receive affection and response, to adapt his powers and interests in common endeavours chosen by the group, to relate to other adults than his parents—these are the elements of the socialization of the self which every human being requires. Like swimming, social relations can best be learned in their own medium—that is, in groups.

Perhaps it is at adolescence when it is most important that this social maturing be made possible in the best possible soil. The group habits of adolescents are now well known. It is also increasingly apparent that such groups exist in and are played upon by a widespread youth peer society, some of whose characteristics are not entirely desirable. It is with such groups that group work can render some of its most valuable service. Recent experiments indicate that group work provides one of the few ways of penetrating the hostile antisocial world of our urban adolescent gang societies.

Activities for children and youth seem to me like the provision of certain elements of social nourishment now lacking in our social soil. They require for success not only a knowledge of individual behaviour, though that is essential, but an intimate knowledge of the behaviour of groups and of the impact upon them of the surrounding society in which they grow.

As we have acquired more insight into this intricate process we have become aware that there are points in which special services are needed in critical situations. We have needed to develop skills to deal with these—the person unable to find and develop the social contacts he wants and needs, the youth unpopular with his fellows and outcast from their groups, the old persons whose family and friends are gone, the isolated adult in the iron lung in a hospital ward, the child crippled by polio and so cut off from normal social contacts, the patient in the ward of a state mental hospital. The urgent necessity for meaningful human contact is all too clear, and the development of appropriate group relations in such circumstances requires the adaptation of what we have learned elsewhere.

The contribution of the group worker to social work and to his society lies, then, in his skill in making various primary-group relations provide for their members heightened social powers, experience in adaptation to the demands of the common enterprise, and enrichment of human contacts and of new interests. All of these are directly related to the ailment of our society with which we began. As our society has come slowly to recognize that many of the social dislocations that call for assistance are in fact the product of society itself, it has increasingly accepted responsibility for the necessary social services.

One further contribution of social work is its part in the administration of the public social services. The modern social services under governmental auspices are characteristic in varying degrees of every industrial society. Social workers have had much to say about the need for such services, about required legislative provisions, about adequacy, and about standards for their proper administration. So long as society regarded such services as arising from emergency or temporary disabilities, society could entrust their administration to private charity. It could maintain the pressure of stigma in the expectation that it would encourage individual enterprise by penalizing pauperism.

Today we are moving toward a different conception. The very

recognition that our kind of society itself produces social disabilities stimulates the realization that society must then make the necessary provisions to deal with the consequences. Florence Kelly used to say of the problem of unemployment, 'Industry must pay its social costs.' Some similar conception is gradually affecting the functions of government in every industrialized country. The very perils of social dislocations with which we deal are often clearly the result not of intrapsychic disturbance or even interpersonal conflict but are a dislocation between a man and his society in which society itself has a large responsibility.

These are *social* products and the remedies must in turn be *social* provisions. As this realization grows the social services slowly cease to to be matters of charity and become matters of right. Society, as Delafield Smith has pointed out, owes to all its members the 'right to life'.[1] It fulfils its obligations in part through the social services.

The contribution of social work as a profession to this great modification of the functions of our society lies at two points. In the first place, although the causes of such dislocations may be in part social they appear in individual human terms in psychological and interpersonal problems. This is why we must have not only adequate income maintenance but also, in many cases, social work services to help clients with the personal results. These may be poor health and little education for migrant children, unemployment resulting from industrial shifts, desertion of wives and children arising out of occupational obsolescence, tensions in changing neighbourhoods, and accompanying adolescent gang fights. The immediate answer for the individual involved must come in part from expert social work service through which caseworkers and group workers can be available to assist in the resulting psychosocial conditions.

During the last twenty-five years has grown the recognition of such social needs, of society's responsibility to meet them, and of some of the ways in which they can constructively be met. Out of these years of effort are gradually emerging the methods, values, and ethics of social work as a profession.

We have recently had expressed for us an outsider's observation of what this new and still somewhat undefined profession is. Delafield Smith, in a recent book growing out of his long experience with the Social Security Board, gives us a lawyer's formulation of what he has observed to be the 'professional idea' of social work.

[1] A. Delafield Smith, *The Right to Life*, University of North Carolina Press, Chapel Hill, 1955.

The professional idea (as distinguished from the police power as he defines it) is positive. 'It involves the proposal to "ride along with" or "run with" the individual in the knowledge that he possesses at base a vital force which, freed as far as possible from whatever blocks or distorts its functioning, is by its very nature or definition a constructive agent. The professional idea proposes to strengthen the capacities of the will of the individual to realize his best goals. It proposes to implement and make constructive use of parental aspirations. It proposes to enable individuals to purchase shelter that meets basic standards of health and decency. It proposes to enable mothers to keep their children when lack of money would cause their abandonment . . . It proposes to provide trained guardians and to see that adoptions are motivated by a concern for the child. It proposes to maintain health in preference to curing illness . . . It proposes to assure the individual of his ability to make higher ground.

The professional idea is seeking to convert weakness into strength. it is proving that the frustrated and defeated individual can be reactivated and that his capacity for constructive and responsible action can be stimulated when there is placed at his disposal the skill, knowledge and strength of someone whose experience has comprehended all that the individual has been up against, and who can use his professional capacities to exalt but not to dominate him. To do this successfully is an art, for it requires . . . seeing his problem as he himself sees it, and then yielding him the use of greater and more specialized knowledge and capacity, while meticulously refraining from any trick or device of self-imposition. The tool that is used is the inspiring effect of intimate human relationships.'[1]

We are all too well aware that the present social welfare services though expanded still do not provide, for all, the 'right to life' in its fullest sense and that they are too often not administered with the full acceptance of the 'professional idea' as defined. It is in large part the achievement of social work that our society as well as our clientele is on the way to 'making higher ground'.

Social responsibility.—The social worker, however, must be concerned not only with the direct provision of his services; his responsibility to society involves him also in certain larger aspects of society's life. Part of this responsibility he must fulfil through working for more adequate social services. Part of it involves the preventive or public health function, the responsibility to contribute as he can

[1] Ibid., pp. 172–73.

to those changes in our social institutions which will reduce social dislocations and make possible healthier and more constructive relations.

A familiar problem can perhaps serve as illustration of such responsibilities. One of the causes of the disruption of social ties and of the creation of socially caused disabilities lies in the mobility of our population. It creates wandering families moving in and out of neighbourhoods, children with part-time or constantly shifting school experience. It destroys old neighbourhood organization and familiar institutions. Churches lose their congregations, stores their customers; real estate values are unstable.

When new ethnic groups move into old neighbourhoods the instability is greater, the shift often more rapid. Established informal leadership is likely to move first. Tensions develop on the streets and in the schools. The sense of a fall in the social scale affects the old inhabitants and they withdraw into isolation or try to make ties in the new areas into which they hope to move. New populations, often from rural sections or sometimes from other areas—Puerto Ricans, Mexicans, displaced persons—have no roots in the new neighbourhoods and often no ties among themselves. The system of adult control over the behaviour of children is either confused or disintegrated. The conflicts between ethnic groups within the area encourage bitter group antagonisms which break out among the teenaged groups especially. Such conditions provide the best breeding grounds for delinquency.

As mobility in our society often is not merely geographical but also social, it has other manifestations. The younger families, established in new, more suburban areas, loosen their ties to parents left behind or change their style of living so that alienation arises between the generations. Youth on the rise dissociates itself from parental control.

These are only a few of the familiar results of one of the major characteristics of our society. We are a population on wheels, but we are also a population climbing upward in standard of living and aspiration for a better class-status and, to a considerable extent, climbing successfully.

What is the relation of social work to these phenomena? We often work in areas where there is mobility of one or both kinds. We see the consequences for individuals, families, and groups. More than the individual is involved, and the answers cannot be found in direct social work services. The society itself is disorganized and uncoagulated. The problem of mobility is one of many in which our answers must lie not primarily in our direct service to clients or groups but in those functions

D

of the social worker which we call 'community organization for social welfare' and, to some extent, in social action.

Our responsibility should lead us to certain definite steps. In the first place, we need to absorb and use more knowledge about the nature of community behaviour. No diagnosis or treatment of any phenomenon is possible without a framework within which to think. To some extent we already have this. We study population movements. We attempt to gauge the changing needs for social welfare services. We provide for the movement of agencies as the needs change. We must, however, go further. Mobility, to be understood, must be seen in terms not only of ecology but of social stratification, of relations between ethnic, racial, and religious groupings, of social aspiration to higher status and the means open to achieve it, of the competitive strain and stress of occupational shift and its consequences, psychological and social.

In other words, the community in such circumstances is our client and as such requires the diagnosis available and appropriate to its life. Beyond this comes treatment. As we observe our present behaviour, we are actually doing several kinds of things. We are not likely to stop the mobility of our population even if it were desirable to do so. However, we are inventing social devices which can mitigate its worst effects. This is perhaps most clearly seen in the so-called 'area projects'. They may involve the organizing of street clubs in changing areas, the co-ordination of local indigenous leadership through co-operative planning, providing service in the newly established communities, or attempting to relate detached group workers to adolescent gangs. Such inventiveness needs to continue to develop new forms of treatment when the client is a disorganized community suffering from a two-way mobility.

More, however, is required. Some aspects of the pathology of communities require not symptomatic treatment but more drastic measures. If we look at what we are doing we will see some clues to what is needed. In the first place, we are tackling on many fronts the problems of those tensions due to racial, ethnic, and, to a lesser, extent, class difference. It is not possible here to detail the methods by which some agencies are working steadily on the problems of intergroup tension and conflict which mobility has brought to their doors. Certainly this was never more urgent than at this particular moment.

One equally basic problem remains—the elimination of slum areas. The slum areas have for generations produced their crop of delinquents. One ethnic group after another may move out of the area. As it becomes assimilated into the total community, its delinquency rate drops. Another group moves in and its rate increases.[1]

The physical elimination of the slum is a highly desirable goal, especially if it can be done in such a way that it does not merely move the slum from one geographical situation to another. However, a slum is more than poor housing and crowded streets. It is psychological and social as well as physical. It is developed in part by the social stratification that labels it in the eyes of the community as the bottom of the heap. A despised ethnic group sinks even further when its place of residence as well as its culture or racial background proclaim it the lowest of the low.

What can be done with this situation? We must work towards certain changes in our social structure. We must eliminate extreme poverty either through a general rise in the standard of living or, for those who cannot benefit from regular economic processes, by special provisions of public assistance and social security. We must keep open and make more available to all the ladders leading to the higher levels of attainment. This we know comes chiefly through educational advantages open to all without discrimination or the discouragement of being continually stigmatized. Perhaps most of all we need to so modify our attitudes and social perspectives that no group in the population feels excluded or looked down upon. These are long range objectives, but to some extent we seem to be moving in that direction.

Social workers know that the stress of a highly competitive society takes its toll not only of those who are thought to fail but of those who seem to succeed. In such a culture the anxiety for achievement will bring strain, emotional and physical, throughout. It is not likely that social work will have much impact on such a major factor. However, if we are aware of the problem and its effect, we are in part equipped at least not to add our own pressures to the competition. In so far, however, as our own values represent human worth and respect for efforts of each to fulfil his own capacities in his own way, we act as moderators of competitive tension and as appreciators of the humane and spiritual values so often ignored in our competitive society.

Goals and values.—Finally, we should not ignore the contribution of the goals and values of social work. I should like to turn to a major current criticism of our society and the relation of social work to it.

Sociologists, historians, theologians, and philosophers point out that

[1] Bertram Beck, 'The Nature of the Delinquency Problem', in *Proceedings of Institute on Team Work for Prevention and Treatment of Juvenile Delinquency*, Western Reserve University, Cleveland, Ohio, June 20–24, 1955.

our society at present suffers from what might be called a disease of the culture, namely, an increasing lack of clarity and agreement as to the meaning of life itself, the place of each person within it, and the hope for our common future or the means of attaining it. These are but symptoms of the fact that mankind, at least Western man, these commentators say, is at present adrift. This affliction may well grow to some extent out of the others we have discussed—the confusion in primary group ties, the dislocations of mobility—but it has other causes also. International conflicts and the possibility of racial extinction deepen the sense of despair. The result, according to our commentators, is an increasing number of people who live in a state of 'anomie', without the clear direction of internalized values. They suffer from what Paul Tillich has called 'the anxiety of meaninglessness'.[1] This affliction is not confined or even concentrated in our clientele. It afflicts us also in many cases, and if it became endemic in our society it would cause that 'failure of nerve' which has preceded the decline and fall of other civilizations. In this realm of values, the answers lie not in the area of facts or of theories about what is but rather in the bases of our own philosophy.

Has the social worker anything to contribute in such a time? Has he convictions that will stand the test of such a social atmosphere? What do we believe which has pertinence today about the meaning of life and the direction of social effort? Obviously, no one can answer for such a large and diverse group as the social work profession. However, values can most often be located in the assumptions that underlie behaviour, and it is here that we may perhaps observe in action some of the values we as social workers hold in common.

Gilbert Murray once summarized what he defined as the religion of democracy: 'The cardinal doctrine of that religion,' he says, 'is the right of every human soul to enter unhindered except by the limitations of its own powers and desires into the full spiritual heritage of the race.'[2] It is this basic tenet, I believe, which motivates us to remove avoidable limitations, to support independence and self-determination, and to encourage the enrichment of life and the development of powers.

As one observes our practice, it seems to me there is another discernible assumption, namely, that in the primary relations of family and intimate group lie the major sources of individual development and of the ultimate consummatory experiences of life. Out of such

[1] Paul Tillich, *The Courage To Be*, Yale University Press, New Haven, 1952, pp. 46–54.
[2] Gilbert Murray, *Tradition and Progress*, Houghton Mifflin Co., Boston, 1922, pp. 29–30.

basic human ties is woven the only sound fabric of society itself, for in them lie the deepest of human satisfactions and the ability to co-operate with others, to give support and effort to the common life without which no democractic society can survive.

If one moves one step back and looks at a community organization worker in a changing neighbourhood, one can see a further assumption, namely, that a human society can be created in which people can work together for common enterprises, in which equality of treatment and mutual respect can be brought about, and in which the larger society can eliminate those social conditions that degrade human life and distort human relations.

Most of us hold one other truth to be self-evident, namely, that our society as a whole must provide for all its members the basic essentials of life, including the means not only to survival but to respect, and freedom of opportunity to expand one's powers in accordance with one's unique needs and capacities.

Although we well know that our practice falls short of these goals, and that at times it is perverted by bureaucracy, or bogged down by narrow technology, the basic values that guide and motivate social workers in direct practice, in preventive social measures, or in social action are a part of that liberal humanitarian tradition that runs through the history and the strivings of our American society. In a day when many seem to suffer from an anxiety of meaninglessness, perhaps one of our greatest contributions to our times is this deepest of our values—our belief in the right of every individual to fulfilment and the responsibility of society to see that it is possible.

These are, of course, not unique. They are the commonly expressed values of our society, but perhaps for us they have a distinctive meaning because we 'work at' them in concrete ways in every act of practice. If we are less naive and less hopeful of immediate results than our professional ancestors, this means only that our increased understanding of the problems of personality and of society have made us more realistic. Our purposes have not changed, only our methods.

It is a characteristic of a fully matured profession that it has not only professional ethics directly related to its practice but that it assumes a responsibility towards its society within its own area of competence. This is, in fact, one of the contributions which each profession makes through its expert advice in its particular field as well as in formulating and incarnating the values and directions appropriate to its functions. The great lawyers, the great doctors, or ministers, or architects are not only primarily expert technicians, though they must be that. They are exemplars, refining and deepening for us all the understanding of the meaning of justice, of the art of healing, of religion, or of beauty. To a lesser extent, every member of a profession is responsible for interpreting to his encompassing society the deepest goals of his profession.

I have no illusions that we shall move our society except by slow degrees towards those views of human relations and social responsibility which are imbedded in our professional values. We are often told these days that we do not have much status. This does not fundamentally concern me. I would not expect that our particular values and goals would bring us acclaim. It is more important that we be sure that our goals are basically sound and that we have sufficient conviction to work for them steadily and intelligently.

Such a professional philosophy held by each of us personally is obviously only a partial view of life. To the thoughtful person and to all who share 'the tragic sense of life' on this beautiful but troubled planet, such a philosophy must rest in a larger context. What is the nature of the cosmos? What is the meaning of history? What is the significance of that which man calls God? What is the essence of good and the nature of evil? Social workers come, as do their clients, from many established faiths, some no doubt of their own invention. Our professional values are necessarily infused with our individual answers to these deeper questions. What I have tried to summarize here is that which I believe we hold *in common* and which relates directly to what we do as social workers. If I am right, however, in this attempt at a summary of our values, it may well be that to hold and act upon such convictions is perhaps one of our best contributions to a society suffering from 'the anxiety of meaninglessness'.

The case for modern man is often stated these days in terms of despair, of withdrawal to old orthodoxies, of the slackening of nerve, and of the sense of impending doom. Here in what we do day by day is, as I see it, a meaning which in a period of confusion and drift could give direction not only to our own efforts but could also strengthen and reaffirm the most essential elements in the faith of Western man and of modern American democracy. We are—among others—the bearers of this tradition. It gives the basic spiritual meaning to our practice and it provides the strong hope that gives courage to our daily efforts.

4

THE SOCIAL WORKER IN THE SIXTIES*

*The Impact of Developing Social Policies on
Established Practices and Attitudes*

E. M. GOLDBERG

RECENTLY I have had the good fortune of experiencing this movement towards greater unity among the specialties of social work at first hand in the Joint Standing Committee of Almoners, Family Caseworkers and Psychiatric Social Workers which met to consider the implications of the Younghusband Report.[1] In our lively discussions one could hear a P.S.W. arguing about the casework needs of the physically handicapped, an almoner outlining how general family casework should and could develop in a health department, and a family caseworker pointing out mental health problems in the community. Any outsider listening, however well informed, would, I am sure, find it extremely difficult to allocate us to our specialties. This, it seems to me, is the outcome of common experiences, an indication that our approach and actual casework practice are becoming more and more alike.

Taking for granted then a common 'generic' approach to the theory and practice of social casework, I want to explore two sets of questions in looking ahead in the 'sixties. First, what are the social policies, needs and administrative frameworks which are likely to shape our work in the coming years?

The Mental Health Act of 1959 is a good guide to the trend in social policy which will be followed in the 'sixties at least. One of its main features is the aim of providing informal admission without any legal formality for almost all persons suffering from mental disorder. For social work the most important element in the Mental Health Act is the

* Published in *The Almoner*, Vol. XIV, No. 3, June, 1961. An address given at the Annual General Meeting of the Institute of Almoners, March 17th, 1961.
[1] Report of the Working Party on Social Workers in the Local Authority Health and and Welfare Services, London, H.M.S.O., 1959.

definition it gives to community care of illness. Section 28 of the National Health Service Act permitted local authorities to provide preventive services, care and after-care for persons suffering from any type of illness in the community. Now with the passing of the Mental Health Act, the government is taking steps in the direction of imposing a duty on local authorities to provide this kind of care. Thus this Act has a special significance for everyone, as it may be regarded as a pilot for extensive social care for all forms of illness and disability. The Younghusband Report with its detailed examination of local authority health and welfare services and its recommendations as to how they may be improved and the necessary staff be trained, is a further step in this direction which has now received government recognition.

We are all aware of the revolution that has taken place in the treatment methods, rehabilitation activities and the general social orientation of mental hospitals. These successes have led to much higher admission and discharge rates of mental hospital patients, and to a great reduction in the average length of stay of the patients which is now less than two months. The more active and optimistic psychiatrists see the possibility of a very great decrease of hospital beds devoted to the care of mental disorder to less than half the existing number. And this opinion has recently been echoed by the Minister of Health. Whether this will really be achieved will depend on the quality of the community care that can be offered. Different types of community care experiments are proceeding in such places as Worthing, Nottingham, Oldham and York; P.E.P. is launching a national enquiry into community mental health services.[1] There is plenty of enthusiasm for learning, experiment and research and no sign of complacency. However, while we can all appreciate the advantages to the community of reducing the burden of patients under hospital care, 'keeping the patient out of hospital' has become an end in itself. This does not appear to be a very rational or justifiable point of view and one to which social workers, I hope, will not fall victim. We need to try and determine the kind of social milieu which can contain the patient in the community without detriment to his treatment or to the health of his family and, similarly, what kind of milieu the patient can be discharged to without endangering his recovery. This implies within the next few years careful observation and 'operational research' in which we as social workers are the essential investigators. The data we acquire in the course of our work if carefully recorded in a uniform way can provide essential information.

[1] 'Community Mental Health Services', *Planning*, Vol. XXVI, No. 447, December, 1960.

Much of the social effort then in the mental health field in the 'sixties will have to go into the provision of various forms of community care for patients, both mentally ill and subnormal, who need not go into hospital at all, as well as those who have spent some time in hospital during acute phases of their illness.

This expansion poses formidable problems as regards the recruitment and training of staff, with which we cannot deal here. However, it is clear that the small minority of professional social workers will have to deploy their resources very carefully. It looks as though many of us will have to forgo the immediate satisfactions of direct casework with patients and their families and instead have to act as consultants, teachers, sorters of problems and co-ordinators, though our basic inspiration will still have to come from direct casework practice, however small the caseloads we can actually carry.

And here it is useful to remember that social casework is only one of the many services (residential and personal) that will have to be enlisted in the care of the sick, the partially recovered and the disabled in the community. The social caseworker of the future may have to act as an interpreter of the needs of the disabled to the community. He will need to help in the activation of community resources on a much greater scale than has even been attempted before: employers' associations, trade unions, churches, clubs, womens' organizations, settlements and other neighbourhood groups will have to play their part if we are in earnest about carrying our mentally disabled in the community.

The need to extend the community care approach to physical illness and disability is obvious. Most almoners, like doctors, are too busy with current patients to be able to follow them up for any length of time after discharge from hospital. Yet there is an accumulating body of evidence that the social care and after-care of the physically ill and disabled is an urgent problem both in economic as well as human terms. For example, Professor Ferguson in Glasgow followed up patients discharged from general hospitals in the West of Scotland.[1] He found that a quarter of men admitted deteriorated seriously within three months of leaving hospital and there was a significant relationship between progress and the quality of the home conditions to which patients were discharged. He also found that only a third complied with advice on management, for example, change of job or diet, which was given them on discharge. A third did not comply at all, and in a third it was doubtful whether they had followed the advice given.

[1] T. Ferguson and A. N. MacPhail, *Hospital and Community*, London, 1954.

Professor Querido[1] in Holland carried out a more complex investigation in which clinical, social and mental factors were taken into account. He found that there was a favourable clinical prognosis in about seventy per cent of the cases investigated, but only in half was this realized—largely because social and psychological factors were militating against recovery. He observed that there was a significant difference in the chance of recovery between patients who had to cope with problems in addition to their physical illness and those who did not.

If we add to the urgent needs for social after-care of the acutely sick, the steadily growing problem of the more or less chronically disabled in late middle and old age, as well as the needs of the blind, the deaf and the permanently physically handicapped, we realize that the scope for community care in the sphere of physical illness and disability is as great and complex as in the sphere of mental disorder. The administrative problems of providing a unified service are almost greater in this field because of the unfortunate split into those services which are administered under Section 28 of the National Health Act in the health departments of local authorities and those for the permanently handicapped, the blind and the deaf, which are provided in the welfare departments under Section 29 of the National Assistance Act, 1948. Thus, if you are suffering from chronic bronchitis and living at No. 37 Smith Street, you may be visited by the social welfare officer of the welfare department, while the boy next door, suffering from tuberculosis, will be visited by the almoner from the health department. I hope that social workers will bring as much pressure as possible to bear to achieve at least close integration—if not amalgamation—of health and welfare services for the handicapped and the sick.

Another administrative problem we shall have to grapple with is that of continuity of care. In the mental health field there are many welcome signs that local authorities and hospital services are experimenting in ways of collaborating, either by formal or informal joint user arrangements—that is to say, by joint appointments of social workers and psychiatrists, by consultation, by hospitals allowing for example mental welfare officers from local authorities to visit patients before discharge and to attend case conferences at the hospitals, and so on. But much still remains to be done in the interest of the patients and their families who often do not fit so neatly into the tripartite arrangements of the health services.

---

[1] A. Querido, 'Forecast and Follow-up. An Investigation into the Clinical, Social and Mental Factors Determining the Results of Hospital Treatment', *British Journal of Preventive and Social Medicine*, Vol. XIII, No. 1, January, 1959.

Similar experiments will be needed in the sphere of physical illness and handicap. For instance, one would hope that local authority workers dealing with the physically disabled can discuss their cases with experienced almoners at hospitals, that advice from hospital consultants and general practitioners will be available to them, and so on.

Finally, the setting in which most of the community care work is to be carried out, the local authority health and welfare departments, poses considerable problems which need to be brought out into the open if they are to be worked out. The introduction of personal and client-centred casework services into the administrative setting of a local authority which is mainly concerned with the provision of more impersonal services for legally defined categories of persons, poses difficulties. For example, the social worker may be concerned with specific needs of individuals and families which may, on occasion, run counter to the provisions or the rules made by the authority for the majority. There are problems of privacy and confidentiality which are not easy to resolve. Consider, for instance, the role of the local councillor who, as an elected representative, is answerable to the public for the conduct of services which of their very nature must be private and confidential. How are we to keep our local councillor informed about and interested in the services we render and yet ensure our clients' right to privacy and confidentiality? How can we instil into employees who may move from department to department the sense of professional secrecy that is more or less taken for granted in medical settings such as hospitals? Much thinking and many discussions will have to take place between administrators and social workers to work out the new roles the local authorities are going to play in relating to the sick and disabled in the community. As had been pointed out in a book on *Sociology in Medicine* by Susser and Watson[1] shortly to appear, these problems have to be recognized as inherent in the complex social structure of bureaucracies and not merely as 'clashes of personalities'. Both administrators and professional workers have social mandates to carry out which occasionally are difficult to reconcile but, as in good clinical practice, correct diagnosis of the problem is the first step towards its resolution.

My second set of questions is concerned with our functions and practices. How can we adapt or enlarge our roles and functions as social workers to meet the challenges posed by the general trend towards community care for the disabled?

[1] M. Susser and W. Watson, *Sociology in Medicine*, Oxford University Press, 1962.

The first necessity is obviously that there should be people to carry out the functions. A look at the distribution of professional social workers shows that the majority of psychiatric social workers and almoners at any rate work in clinical or hospital settings for which their training explicitly qualifies them. Amongst almoners and P.S.W.s there has been a gradual movement towards community care during the last few years.

The proportion of P.S.W.s in mental hospitals to P.S.W.s in local authorities is now four (220) to one (50),[1] the equivalent proportion of almoners in hospitals and local authority settings is 17 (1,000) to one (60). Hospital team work under the leadership of the consultant is a satisfying professional experience for medical social workers. They might occasionally criticize and kick against some of the hierarchical features of the hospital system but I have gained the impression that most almoners feel comfortable and happy within the great healing traditions of general and particularly teaching hospitals. There is a grave shortage of almoners in most hospitals so in their case as well as in that of P.S.W.s to take up community work means robbing Peter to pay Paul. Anyway, let us be frank: to venture forth into a health department of a local authority, perhaps as the only almoner among a group of administrators, health visitors, and social welfare officers, catching an occasional fleeting glimpse of the deputy medical officer of health, without a room for interviewing, private telephone or filing cabinet, is not a very tempting prospect. Still, we shall have to face the problem of priorities, realizing that the supply of professionally trained social workers in the health field will remain limited for many years to come. There can be no easy or single answer and over the next years I can only visualize the gradual working out of a number of compromises which will make the boundaries between hospital and local authority services more and more flexible and suited to the individual needs of patients and their families. I can also visualize a gradual broadening of the functions of hospital almoners in three directions: in the type of casework carried out about which I will have more to say; in their greater participation in the training of medical students so that succeeding generations of doctors may have a much clearer grasp and understanding of the social components in illness; and in the development of close collaboration with colleagues in the local authority health departments.

Let us consider the casework functions of hospital almoners which were set out so brilliantly by Jean Snelling in her paper given in the

[1] Association of Psychiatric Social Workers, Annual Report, 1960.

series 'New Trends in Social Work' at the London School of Economics in the autumn of 1959.[1] She defined nine such functions from which I select the three core ones: (1) helping patients with social problems which impede medical care; (2) studying and assessing patients' social situations to help the doctors in diagnosis; (3) social work with patients in illness management, for instance helping them with their fear of hospitals, of illness, and of death.

There seems to exist another specific function which may be covered by Miss Snelling's point (1)—but which needs stating explicitly: help towards rehabilitation. Most almoners are in fact involved in this function which may be primarily one of communication with the general practitioner, the local authority, the disablement resettlement officer, the patient's family, to ensure that the plans so carefully worked out in the hospital are understood and translated into reality.

The formulation which I found most thought-provoking, however, was Miss Snelling's third function—that of illness management. She argues that the social worker rather than the doctor would be more able to deal with these problems because the doctor's function is to fight illness rather than to care for sick people. In his job of 'attacking the illness' he may not have much time or feeling left for the care function which almoners are in a good position to supplement.

Some doctors agree with this division of function. They stress the matter of priorities, saving life, the time factor and the shortage of doctors, pointing out that in the future there will be fewer, not more, doctors. Some almoners have observed certain interesting stereotypes which also support Miss Snelling's argument. Patients often feel that doctors have no time and almoners all the time in the world; they feel that because so much depends on the good powerful doctor they in turn must live up to his expectations of a good patient and show their bravest front and not admit their fears to him, but that they can 'let their hair down' to the almoner who is socially nearer to them and less awe-inspiring. I have also listened to patients' reminiscences during a small follow-up study and have been impressed with their inability to ask any questions at all while in hospital, and it has turned out not infrequently that the person who had the most intimate contact and learnt most of the patient's uncertainties was the medical student who might have spent many hours with him.

Sometimes I wonder whether there is some element of collusion between doctors and social workers in this sphere of illness manage-

[1] Jean Snelling, 'Social Work within Medical Care', *The Almoner*, Vol. XV, No. 3, June, 1962.

ment. The doctors tend more and more to regard the social workers as the experts in regard to social and psychological problems. This absolves the doctors from the necessity of tacking these difficult and intractable components of illness and enables almoners to do worthwhile and interesting casework and feel themselves part of the therapeutic team. Where do I stand? Let me admit that as a person who perhaps foolishly still nourishes the fantasy of the future doctor seeing his patient as a whole person, I feel deeply uneasy about this division of functions which splits the patient into a physical organism, a case, an illness to be dealt with by the doctor; and a person with social and psychological needs to be attended to by the almoner. It brings into the open an issue which doctors and social workers will have to explore together. Does the ever-increasing specialization and scientific precision in medicine demand the hospital physician's exclusive concentration on particular aspects of disease and is our hankering after the holistic approach unrealistic? Is Miss Snelling's proposition the sensible, workable compromise? Or is there an alternative: to reshape medical training so that doctors consider it their job to care for patients as persons who are beset by fears and anxieties. Some physicians would then carry out the functions of illness management themselves, thus freeing almoners to devote time to problems which hospital doctors are unable to reach, namely the environmental and social problems which lie outside the hospital confines within the patient's family, his work situation, his community setting and so on.

Let us examine some of these functions outside the hospital within their historical context.

Insights and practices derived mainly from dynamic psychology have led some social caseworkers to concentrate very much on the individual client as the product of his early relationships; they have also led to a heightened awareness of the unconscious and irrational elements in people's conduct and to a corresponding decreasing interest in the social situation which impinges on our clients. This in turn has resulted in a patient- or client-centred form of therapy in which the searchlight is focused on the past and the patient's inner world rather than on the present and the external world. A further corollary of this development is the predominant use of the office interview.

I believe that these trends were to some extent inevitable in the evolution of social casework. When we rediscovered in our own work (and not simply by reading psychoanalytic textbooks) that the child was the father to the man and that even such gross social problems as chronic debts could rarely be ascribed exclusively or even mainly to the operation of economic factors or to ignorance of social services available, but to powerful emotional forces working *within* the individual concerned, it is understandable that we applied ourselves with fervour and enthusiasm to the exploration and modification of these inner forces. It is even more understandable if one considers that the same period of time saw the development of the Welfare State and the emergence of the affluent society which abolished many, though by no means all, forms of gross poverty and social injustice with which our predecessors had to struggle. But do some of us tend to become lost in the ever deeper exploration of the powerful emotional drives that shape our clients' destinies and to ignore the present forces, psychological, social and economic which continually interact with these inner drives and which are also highly complex, dynamic and worthy of study? Are we in some danger of impoverishing our potentially unique contribution to social diagnosis and therapy, inviting the now familiar attacks of being the poor man's pseudo-psychiatrist and, last but not least, of sometimes failing our clients?

I should like to propose that, having by now securely incorporated into the theory and practice of social casework the basic tenets of dynamic psychology, we might usefully rediscover the social environment in which our clients move, not as a static framework but as a dynamic process continually interacting with inner personal forces. This may well become our main practical and theoretical task in the coming years.

I should like to illustrate this reappraisal of our clients' social environment as a dynamic force by discussing the study of the home environment, family interaction and the work situation.

The study of the home environment necessitates consideration of our old discarded friend, the home visit. May I recall some of the arguments against it? A home interview interferes with the aims of therapeutic discussion. Children may come home from school and interrupt, something may be boiling over on the stove, the tally man may call, the telephone may ring and so on. By visiting, social workers intrude upon their clients, entering their homes as of right, without giving them any choice in the matter. Here we detect unpleasant memories of the days when determined ladies looked at mattresses and 'inspected' the home, thus denying their clients' rights to privacy. The effort of keeping an appointment at a certain place is seen as a valuable part of treatment. It is argued that the office interview makes for a more professional relationship; the environment is more neutral; it is easier for the client to detach himself from the daily round and to review his personal and family life in a new light. Most importantly, it saves the caseworker's time. The theoretical argument maintains that what matters most in social casework is what people feel about things rather than what these things are really like. It is more important—some of our colleagues tell us—to learn what Mrs X feels about her home than what it actually looks like.

But have we recently over-emphasized the advantages of the office interview and tended to ignore some of the advantages of observing our clients in their natural habitat? First of all, thinking of the mental health field, some of the people who need our help most—the severely withdrawn or depressed patients and their families—may not have the energy or initiative to seek us, we will have to go to them. Here, incidentally, we touch upon another piece of orthodoxy in our practice: that we can only help, or should attempt to help, people who feel the need. This would immediately exclude many problem families, many severely disturbed and subnormal people who desperately need our help though they may not know it or deny it; and probation officers, for example, could not claim to do social casework because their functions are usually imposed on their clients to begin with. It is true, of course, that, while we need to reach out to some of our clients because they are not able to ask for our help, we always respect their right to refuse our services and try to stimulate their co-operation. But, if we insist on consulting room practices, on rigid appointment systems, and on our clients seeking our help only when they are ready for it, then we rob ourselves of our flexibility as social workers. We could no longer be a sort of half-way house between the clinic or institution in which we work and the community, available to our clients in a variety of ways and situations, and we would thus narrow our professional functions.

And what about the theoretical argument that what Mrs X feels about her home matters more than what it actually looks like? Are they not both important—the reality and the feeling about it?

Is there not here a confusion between casework and psychotherapy? In intensive psychotherapy or psychoanalysis people project their feelings and experiences on to the therapist's screen; gradually over the months and years the distortions may be perceived and worked through and both the therapist and the patient may finally arrive at an approximately true picture of reality as it is. In the context of social casework, which is less concerned with deep personality changes than with modifying attitudes within a social situation, the appraisal of the social reality which includes the social, psychological and cultural milieu may be of crucial diagnostic and therapeutic significance. I find it a very great help to experience what Mrs X's home looks like. It tells me a great many things about her personality, her likes and dislikes, her home-making qualities and some of her aspirations. I can learn much by observing what goes on, whether they be interruptions by children coming home from school or visitors dropping in. The important point is that the home visit is a different kind of technique, yielding different kinds of information from the office interview. It involves as much skill, and usually more if several family members are present; it can be just as planned a piece of casework, in which similar forces of interaction between client and worker are called into play. But there is an added social dimension for us to observe, the interaction between our client and his social environment. Nor need the client feel inferior or 'inspected'. I take it for granted that home visits in 1961 will be by appointment and mutual consent. Indeed, some people have argued that the clients may feel less at the mercy of the worker and the somewhat overawing agency in which she functions if they are the hosts and can give something in return, even if it be only a cup of tea.

Some colleagues have argued that health visitors could obtain home reports if need be to supplement the caseworker's findings. This view suggests an unreal dichotomy between a static physical environment and a dynamic personal reality; whereas in fact the social situation and the personality are in continuous interaction, and it is this interaction we, as social workers, are mainly concerned with and must try to observe. The main point at issue is—when are such home visits indicated, and under what circumstances do they provide better diagnostic and therapeutic opportunities than office interviews? Only experiment will tell—let me mention two.

One is the work carried out by a medical social worker, Jane Paterson, when she was working in a comprehensive maternal and child care programme at Harvard University School of Public Health. Some of her findings were reported in *The Almoner* under the title 'The Use of the Home Visit in Present-Day Social Work.[1]' In this project experiences of families during a first pregnancy were observed. In the course of it fifty home visits were paid and Miss Paterson asked herself whether the home visit had any value and what it adds to the contact with the client in the agency setting. Very shortly, her findings were that seeing the parents in the home setting often provided new factual information which helped to round out the impressions formed

[1] Jane Paterson and Florence Cyr, 'The Use of the Home Visit in Present-Day Social Work', *The Almoner*, Vol. XIII, No. 7, October, 1960.

at the clinic interview. In some cases new insight into the family situation was gained and in many cases seeing the home itself and the standards of home-making shed light on the personalities of the parents and their life together. For example, the way they talked with each other, the way they shared the baby care, the ways in which they responded to their joint responsibility. She adds that the contribution made by grandmothers and other relatives could gradually be seen as an assistance or a complication, and that as a result of what the worker saw and heard at the home visit, future plans for the support of the parents and their individual or joint responsibilities could be worked out in conjunction with other members of the team. Miss Paterson found that the home interview did not militate against the professional relationship but actually strengthened it, and she concluded that the added knowledge gained from the home visit resulted in a social diagnosis more useful to other members of the clinic team and in a more effective total treatment plan.

A similar kind of experience which enlarged the social diagnosis and occasionally instituted new treatment plans was gained from a small follow-up study of coronary patients carried out by an almoner and a psychiatric social worker to ascertain how patients had settled down at work and at home, what their residual problems were, and how much help they and their relatives had derived from advice on management given at the hospital. These home visits were long interviews in which wives were almost always present and they ranged over the patient's life and work as well as his present situation. The full reports were passed on unedited to the consultant concerned who apparently found them most illuminating and surprising. For example, he learned that patients did not understand how nitrite should be taken, often firmly believing that it was a dangerous and habituating drug; that most patients had been too anxious to ask about the nature of their illness or to take in the information when it was given; that their wives had hardly ever felt able to approach the doctors and, at times, not even the sister; and that, on the whole, the wives were in ignorance as to what kind of management had been prescribed for work and leisure and what generally to expect. At the same time both patients and their families were deeply grateful to the hospital. Nor had the general practitioners made good their deficiencies in the year following the discharge from hospital.

It is doubtful whether these attitudes would have been expressed so freely and naturally in the hospital environment, nor would one have gained such a complete picture from seeing patients without their wives. For example, one patient who was doing extremely well and had gone back to his full-time job was prone to deny any ill-effects of his illness, and his wife indicated that she needed to be present at the interview to correct this rosy picture.

What these home visits taught both the social workers and the doctors most vividly was the interaction between (a) the illness, (b) the personality of the patient and (c) his social environment, the most significant feature of the last being the nature of the support received from the family and the suitability and significance of the job. The interaction of these factors had never stood out so clearly in hospital interviews. There was, for example, the patient who, though organically quite well, seemed unable to move even a few steps and complained that he was in pain when he ate. The home visit revealed a sick, painfully thin wife suffering from anorexia and nervous dyspepsia who clearly regarded herself as the patient of the family with whom the ex-coronary had to compete.

As a result of this small follow-up a leaflet on the use and function of nitroglycerine was produced and the consultant also instituted a final follow-up interview with the patient *and* his wife in which he tried to ensure that both understood the nature of the illness and its management and he encouraged them to ask questions freely. It seems as though these home reports had added a new dimension to the picture the consultant had of his patients.

Home visits afford unique opportunities for seeing the family functioning as a group and for working with several members of the family at the same time. This brings me to another aspect in which we might reassess our practice—the awareness of family interaction. Knowledge is growing slowly about the ways in which individual needs and role expectations interlock and how they result in a specific balance of forces in any given family. An awareness of these forces should inform both social diagnosis and treatment; work with one member of the family will not only affect his attitudes, needs and expectations but, in turn, the needs and expectations of those near him—and hence, the balance of forces in the family. Thus the treatment aims we pursue with one individual must either be compatible with the needs of the other members or, where this is not possible, the others must also be helped to a new adjustment.

Consider for example the case of the middle-aged married coronary patient who revealed considerable marital problems to the almoner and painted his wife as a cold and non-understanding person unable to respond to the needs of an invalid husband who was no longer the active leader in the home. From this man's early childhood history it was clear that this image of a cold hostile wife was carried over from his feelings about his own mother and sister, but it was difficult to work through this without the opportunities for reality testing which joint interviews with the wife would have provided. In such a joint interview the wife might have learned something about the nature of her husband's fears. Her responses might have indicated to the husband that his image of his wife as a cold unsympathetic person was not justified, and the worker might have helped him to see that these feelings belonged to his past experiences. A discussion about altered roles might have ensued in which one could have helped the wife towards an adjustment to a husband no longer the active, efficient centre of the home. What happened in actual fact was that this man felt so guilty about the things he had said about his wife that he could not allow the worker to see her, and after another interview he never reappeared in the almoner's office though still attending the out-patient department of the hospital.

In child guidance, workers have in the past concentrated on the mother-child relationship and have tended to work with mothers as though fathers had no part to play. Yet now that I have occasion to deal with the families of mentally very sick young men I am struck by the magnitude of the father-son problems. Sometimes the following chain of events can be observed: the patient may have attended a child guidance clinic and much-needed casework may have been carried out with the mother who was deeply involved in her child's illness—but the father was left outside, anxious, resentful, often described as useless and inadequate by the mother and not interested in his children. The father proceeds to react with added scorn and contempt for the son who cannot stand up to the stresses of life, forever protected, fussed and hustled by his mother. Serious disagreements arise over the management of the sick boy's growing inertia. The son, as he drifts from job to job, feels that the gap between his performance and his father's, who has kept his foreman's job for twenty odd years, becomes unbridgeable until in despair he finally gives up completely.

Or the father may indeed be the one positive force on whom to build one's main casework effort. I am thinking of a case where the mother was an ineffective woman, prone to severe depressions when she could not manage her children or her housework. The husband, who was on shift work, did a great deal in the house, often looked after the children and was the stable force in the home. But most of the social workers who had attempted to help had concentrated on Mrs X, trying to ease her burden by arranging holidays for her and the children, or school meals, without consulting the father. He often withheld consent to quite reasonable practical suggestions because he felt himself to be ignored and his role not appreciated. When at last a family caseworker appeared on the scene who saw both parents and made it his business to enlist the father's help and explain his wife's condition to him it was quite easy to get his consent for various forms of assistance.

Sometimes our very success in treatment with one member of the family may upset the balance of the family equilibrium. I am thinking of work with alcoholics. Edgar Myers and others[1,2] have shown that alcoholics are prone to marry rather energetic, nurse-type of wives who like responsibility and may enjoy having a dependent and irresponsible 'child' for whom they can care efficiently. Time and again it has been found that once the husband overcomes his alcoholism his wife either becomes depressed or ill herself or manages by subtle means to undermine the improvement so that the man will start drinking again. The same can apply to work in marital situations. If a rather dependent ineffective child-wife who has been cosseted and protected by her father-like husband becomes as a result of treatment more mature and independent, she will look for different qualities in her partner and her husband may find himself rejected in his accustomed role.

The more I work with family problems the more I realize that work with one spouse alone almost invariably leads to distortion of the role the other spouse plays, and however skilled we are, it happens only too easily that we may gang up with one partner against the other.

If we have a sensitive awareness of complementary needs and roles in a family situation we may, on occasion, even desist from doing any casework at all. I am reminded of a marriage which was satisfying to both partners although built on mutual neurotic needs. An immature, dependent man, a permanent invalid who had lacked maternal love in his childhood, had some of his needs fulfilled by his maternal self-sacrificing wife. She, on the other hand, in order to satisfy her needs of emulating a much admired father had to keep her husband a dependent child, thus preventing him from ever growing up emotionally. Although this marital relationship was determined by childhood fixations, it provided substitute satisfactions and enabled these two people to lead useful and even happy lives, though as individuals they

[1] Edgar Myers, 'Alcoholics and their Families', *Case Conference*, Vol. I, No. 6, October, 1954.

[2] Betty Knock, 'The Marital Problems of Neurotic Patients in a Mental Hospital', *Case Conference*, Vol. I, No. 10, February, 1955.

both were emotionally disabled.[1] Were they in need of treatment?

One final point on family interaction. When I refer to the study of the family environment I do not only include the conscious or unconscious interaction of personal factors but, also, the understanding of social roles and norms current in society. A body of knowledge is slowly accumulating. In order to make this knowledge available to social caseworkers in a meaningful form we need to develop a sociology for social workers which attempts to link together facts about social structure with the evolving knowledge about the dynamics of family life, the work situation and processes of communication.

Finally, there is yet another sphere in which we need to broaden our function and learn a great deal more and that is the world of work. We are all deeply interested in the maternal role and problems of child care. We have paid little attention to paternal functions and to the study of the spheres in which men move for the greater part of their lives—their work. For example, many of the young mental patients I meet experience great difficulties in their work roles. Often intensive efforts have gone into industrial rehabilitation in the hospital only to be undone by the patient's subsequent inability to find suitable work or to continue to derive inspiration from work. Specialist services are available at the Ministry of Labour, but more knowledge on our part is required if we are to help our colleagues at the Ministry of Labour with adequate interpretation of our patients' needs. In the field of middle-aged disability I have been impressed with the great social and psychological significance of work. Feeling useful and adequate at work seems deeply linked with self-respect and self-acceptance in men and hence with tolerable functioning. Continually I have felt handicapped by the lack of actual concrete knowledge of how industrial processes work, what factory life is really like and what kind of demands are made on different types of workers. I have often wondered whether I would be able to help both the young and the old more if I had a more concrete picture of the supports and stresses their work situations contain. This knowledge will all the more be needed in the years to come. Rehabilitation of the physically and mentally ill and disabled will become a major part of our activities, and retirement problems of an increasing proportion of our population will loom large in our work.

This brings me to the end of my speculations about possible growing points of social work in the 'sixties. More of us will be concerned with

[1] E. M. Goldberg, 'The Normal Family—Myth and Reality', *Social Work*, Vol. XVI, No. 1, January, 1959. Reprinted in *Social Work with Families, Readings in Social Work*, No. 1, Compiled by Eileen Younghusband, George Allen and Unwin, 1965.

the community care of the sick, the partially recovered and the disabled. Many of us will have to help out as consultants and in disseminating what knowledge we have. We have considered some of the administrative difficulties that will face us in the near future—the problems of continuity of care and those inherent in the structure of local authority services.

We have also examined our functions and practices. I have suggested that whether we work in the hospital or the community we need to pay more attention to the social environment in which our patients live. We looked afresh at the use of the home visit, the complexities of family interaction and the roles of men at home and at work.

It seems to me then that if we can learn to combine our understanding of individual and social forces we shall make a distinct contribution as social workers in the coming years.

5

FAMILY DIAGNOSIS: VARIATIONS IN THE BASIC VALUES OF FAMILY SYSTEMS*

FLORENCE ROCKWOOD KLUCKHOHN

FOR many years my own interest has been centred on the variations of the quite universal institution commonly called The Family. And the still broader perspective has been the variations in basic value—value orientations—found both between cultures and within cultures. Therefore, it is from this point of view that I wish to approach the problems of diagnosing and treating disturbances in family relations.

Psychologically speaking, it is well known that the developing personalities of children are greatly affected by the kinds of relationships they have with a mother, a father, and siblings. Sometimes, but not very often, in the analysis of family patterns made in this country the influences of grandparents and collateral relatives are considered. But even when these are considered, not much attention has been given to the differing effects of culturally variable family patterns upon the relationships themselves and the kinds of personalities which result from them.

In a research programme now in progress under the joint direction of Dr John Spiegel and myself, an attempt is being made so to integrate the concepts of psychological and cultural theory that there will be a better understanding of the interaction of the cultural and the psychological aspects of the socialization process.[1]

Specifically, this research is centred on an analysis of the interrelatedness of factors that contribute to the emotional 'health' and 'illness' of families. The focus of attention in the research is always the family and not the individual, because we believe that many, if not most, of the disturbances seen in individual members of families are in some sense a product of the disturbances in the whole network of personal interrelations in the families. So much is this the case that we

* Published in Social Casework, Vol. XXXIX, Nos. 2–3, February/March, 1958.
[1] This research is a project in the Laboratory of Social Relations of Harvard University. It is sponsored and financed by the National Institute of Mental Health.

expected that improvement in the mental health of the member defined as 'sick' would very frequently be countered by an outbreak of disturbance elsewhere in the family system. This is to say that very often the illness of one member, particularly a child, has functional significance for family equilibrium. The results thus far obtained seem to be in agreement with this expectation.

One of the factors we wished to give special attention to was the cultural one, or—I would prefer to say—the value orientation factor. We were concerned with finding out both what kinds of strains are common to families and particular cultures or subcultures and what additional ones are to be expected when a family is in process of acculturation.

Because of this interest, and others that there is not time to go into here, we developed a research design that would control much of the variability that is inevitably found by the therapist who usually takes families 'as they come'. Very briefly the design was as follows. A total caseload of eighteen families, half of which could be defined as 'sick' and half as 'well' or 'normal', was decided upon. We felt that, even with a fairly large staff, more families than this number could not be handled.

The 'sick' family cases were obtained through a hospital and medical centre concerned solely with children. Thus, the sickness of the family was in the first instance defined by the family itself or those who had made the referral because of the illness of a child. We limited the age range of the children to four to thirteen years for we did not, at this stage of our investigation, want to complicate the research with the special problems of adolescence.

The so-called 'well' families were selected from the wider metropolitan community. In most instances the contacts with them were arranged through public health and social agencies. In two cases the co-operation of families was gained through personal connections of members of the research team.

The definition of a family as 'well' is, of course, a complicated matter. Our first criterion was simply the fact that the family itself and others in contact with its children (teachers and doctors, for example) did not consider any of the children sufficiently disturbed to be referred for treatment. Another criterion of our own making was the seeming ability of a family to handle its problems—and certainly no family is without problems—without using one or two of its members as targets for a projection of unresolved and denied tensions. It would take too long to discuss in detail the other differences that were either expected or discovered. Let me say only that in our caseload, as it was finally arranged, we have really a continuum from what we have designated as 'sick' to what we call 'well' but the dividing line is clearly enough marked to keep cases on one side or the other.

The next requirement we set was a selection of families, both 'sick' and 'well', by ethnic background. The three groups selected were so-called Old American, Irish-American, and Italian-American. In all cases every effort was made to have these ethnic strains pure and, for the most part, we achieved our goal. We wished further, in the cases of the Irish- and Italian-Americans, to have families with American-born parents and foreign-born grandparents. We were not entirely successful in meeting this requirement. In part the reason was that another of our require-ments handicapped such a selection. This was that some, if not all, grandparents should be in the area and available for interviewing.

Other requirements, which led many of those who were helping us select the cases to say that we could never find the sample, were these: The families had to have more than one but fewer than eight children; there could be no examples of broken homes; psychotic or border-line psychotic (atypical) children and children with known or suspected organic impairments (brain damage, for example) were not to be in-cluded; and, finally, all families should come from the social class range of upper-lower to lower-middle class.

For the most part, our sample accords with all these criteria. We have also been able to meet the very basic requirement that in the handling of the 'sick' cases the father, the mother, and the child are all seen with equal regularity. In addition some interviews and observa-tions have been made in the homes. In the 'well' families all interview-ing has been in the homes, and all members have been observed. In a few instances the psychological testing (another of the research require-ments) of some members of 'well' families has been done in the clinic.

This was the sample which was so arranged as to allow us to test fairly well our hypothesis that variations in the value orientations of the families of subcultures make for differences in types of problems found in family relations and in the motivation for treatment.

But when I speak of variation in value orientations I have reference to a particular theory about such variation which has been evolved over a period of many years from fairly continuous cross-cultural research. It is necessary to present this theory in summary outline before more can be said, even illustratively, about either our expectations or our findings.

In recent decades, anthropologists notably (but others, too, such as the philosophers, F. S. C. Northrup and Charles Morris) have made us increasingly aware of the fact that although human beings the world over may face many of the same basic life problems, they do not, either cognitively or affectively find the same solutions for them. Moreover, basic values are not superficial phenomena. The value orientations (the term I prefer) of a people are deeply rooted, are mainly unconscious, and are also so pervasive that they markedly affect the patterns of behaviour and thought of a people in all areas of activity. Let me quote a statement from Clyde Kluckhohn:

'There is a "philosophy" behind the way of life of every individual and of every relatively homogeneous group at any given point in their histories. This gives, with varying degrees of explicitness or implicitness, some sense of coherence or unity to living both in cognitive and affective dimensions. Each personality gives to this "philosophy" an idiosyncratic colouring, and creative individuals will markedly reshape it. However, the main outlines of the fundamental values, existential assumptions, and basic abstractions have only exceptionally been created out of the stuff of unique biological heredity and peculiar life experience. The underlying principles arise out of, or are limited by, the givens of biological human nature and the universalities of social interaction. The specific formulations is ordinarily a cultural product. In the immediate sense, it is from the life-ways which constitute the designs for living of their community or tribe or region or socioeconomic class or nation or civilization that most individuals derive their "mental-feeling outlook" '.[1]

The anthropologist, dealing with quite different cultures the world around, has concerned himself mostly with a demonstration of the often dramatic differences between cultures. What I wish now to present is a classification of values and some ideas about variation which allow us to analyse both this kind of difference and the other kind which I call intracultural variation. In outlining the theory I shall use illustrations from the Spanish-American culture to which I have devoted much time and still others far removed from the three groups that are the main concern of the research I have described. Subsequently I shall give illustrations of the application of the theory in our current research.

A CLASSIFICATION OF VALUE ORIENTATIONS*

Three major assumptions underlie both the classification system of value orientations and the conceptualization of aspects of variation in value orientations.

[1] Clyde Kluckhohn and others, 'Values and Value-Orientations in the Theory of Action', in *Toward a General Theory of Action*, Talcott Parsons and Edward A. Shils (eds), Harvard University Press, Cambridge, 1952, Part 4, Chapter 2, pp. 209–10.

* For a fuller discussion of this classification scheme and the theory of variation in value

First, it is assumed that *there is a limited number of common human problems for which all peoples at all times must find some solution*. This is the universal aspect of value orientations because the common human problems to be treated arise inevitably out of the human situation.

But however universal the problems, the solutions found for them are not the same; hence the next consideration is the degree of relativity or, better, the range of variability. The second assumption is that *while there is variability in solutions of all the problems, it is neither limitless nor random but is definitely variable within a range of possible solutions*.

The third assumption, which provides the key to the later analysis of variation in value orientations, is that *all variants of all solutions are in varying degrees present in all societies at all times*. Thus, every society has, in addition to its dominant profile of value orientations, numerous *variant* or *substitute profiles*. And in both the dominant and the variant profiles, there is always a *rank ordering* of ¡value orientations emphases rather than a single emphasis.

Five problems have been tentatively singled out as the crucial ones common to all human groups. These problems are stated here in the form of questions, and in each case there is a parenthetical designation of the name that will be used hereafter for the range of orientations relating to the question:

1. What is the character of innate human nature? (*Human-Nature* Orientation)

2. What is the relation of man to nature (supernature)? (*Man-Nature* Orientation)

3. What is the temporal focus of human life? (*Time* Orientation)

4. What is the modality of human activity? (*Activity* Orientation)

5. What is the modality of man's relationship to other men? (*Relational* Orientation).

The ranges of variability suggested as a testable conceptualization of the variation in the value orientations are given in Table I [on next page].

orientations see two articles by the author, 'Dominant and Substitute Profiles of Cultural Orientations'[1] and 'Dominant and Variant Value Orientations'.[2]

A still more complete version of the theory, as well as the results of testing it in five cultures, appears in *Variations in Value Orientations*.[3]

[1] Florence Rockwood Kluckhohn, 'Dominant and Substitute Profiles of Cultural Orientations: Their Significance for the Analysis of Social Stratification', *Social Forces*, Vol. XXVIII, Nov. 4, 1950, pp. 276–293.

[2] ——, 'Dominant and Variant Value Orientations', in *Personality in Nature, Society, and Culture*, Clyde Kluckhohn and Henry A. Murray (eds), Alfred A. Knopf, New York, 2nd ed., 1953, pp. 342–57.

[3] ——, Fred L. Stordtbeck, and others, *Variations in Value Orientations*, Row, Peterson & Co., Evanston, Illinois, 1961.

Table 1

Innate Human Nature	Evil	Neutral	Mixture of Good and Evil	Good
	Mutable-Immutable	Mutable-Immutable		Mutable-Immutable
Man's Relation to Nature and Supernature	Subjugation to Nature	Harmony with Nature		Master over Nature
Time Focus	Past	Present		Future
Modality of Human Activity	Being	Being-in-Becoming		Doing
Modality of Man's Relationship to Other Men	Lineal	Collateral		Individualistic

NOTE: Since each of the orientations is considered to be independently variable, the arrangement in columns of sets of orientations is only the accidental result of this particular diagram. All combinations are considered to be possible. For example, a Doing Activity orientation may be combined with a Mastery-over-Nature position and Individualism, as it is in dominant American culture; or, as one finds in Navaho Indian culture, it may be in combination with a first order Harmony-with-Nature position and Collaterality.

1. *Human Nature Orientation*. To the question of what innate *human-nature* is, there are the three logical divisions of Evil, Good and Evil, and Good. Yet it may be argued that the category of Good *and* Evil is not one but two categories. There certainly is a significant difference between the view that human nature is simply neutral and the view of it as a mixture of the good and bad. Moreover, the subprinciples of mutability and immutability increase the basic threefold classification to six possibilities. Human nature can, for example, be conceived to be— Evil and unalterable or Evil and perfectible; as Good and unalterable or Good and corruptible; as an invariant mixture of the Good and Evil or as a mixture subject to influence.

Few will disagree that the orientation inherited from Puritan ancestors and still strong among many Americans is that of a basically Evil but perfectible *human nature*. According to this view constant control and discipline of the self are required if any real goodness is to be achieved, and the danger of regression is always present. But some in the United States today, perhaps a growing number, incline to the view that human nature is a mixture of the Good and Evil. These would say that although control and effort are certainly needed, lapses can be understood and need not always be severely condemned. This latter definition of basic human nature would appear to be a more common one among peoples of the world, both literate and nonliterate, than the one held to in the historical past of this country. Whether there are any total societies committed to the definition of human nature as immutably Good is to be doubted. Yet the position is a possible one, and it certainly is found as a variant definition within societies.

2. *Man-Nature (-Supernature) Orientation.* The three-point range of variation in the *man-nature* orientation-Subjugation to Nature, Harmony with Nature, and Mastery over Nature – is too well known from the works of philosophers and culture historians to need much explanation. Mere illustrations will demonstrate the differences between the conceptions.

Spanish-American culture in the American Southwest gives us an example of a very definite Subjugation-to-Nature orientation. The typical Spanish-American sheep herder in a time as recent as fifteen years ago believed firmly that there was little or nothing a man could do to save or protect either land or flocks when damaging storms descended upon them. He simply accepted the inevitable. In Spanish-American attitudes towards illness and death one finds the same fatalism. 'If it is the Lord's will that I die, I shall die', is the way they express it, and many a Spanish-American has refused the services of a doctor because of this attitude.

If the conceptualization of the man-nature relationship is that of Harmony, there is no real separation between man, nature, and supernature. One is simply an extension of the other and the conception of wholeness derives from their unity. This orientation, little understood in this country since it is a third order one, seems to have been the dominant one in many periods of Chinese history, and it is strongly evident in Japanese culture at the present time as well as historically. It is also the orientation attributed to the Navaho Indians by Clyde Kluckhohn.

The Mastery-over-Nature position is the first order one of most Americans. Natural forces of all kinds are to be overcome and put to the use of human beings. Rivers everywhere are spanned with bridges; mountains have roads put through and around them; new lakes are built, sometimes in the heart of a desert; old lakes get partially filled in when additional land is needed for building sites, roads, or airports; the belief in man-made medical care for the control of illness and the lengthening of life is strong to an extreme; and all are told early in life that 'the Lord helps those who help themselves'. The view in general is that it is a part of man's duty to overcome obstacles; hence the great emphasis upon technology.

3. *Time Orientation.* The possible cultural interpretations of the temporal focus of human life break easily into the three-point range of Past, Present, and Future. Far too little attention has been given to the full range of major variations in the *time* orientation.

Obviously, every society must deal with all the three time problems; each one has its conceptions of the past, the present, and the future. Where societies differ is in the rank order emphasis given to each, and a very great deal can be told about the particular society or part of a society being studied, much about the direction of change within it can be predicted, if one knows what the rank order emphasis is.

Illustrations of the variations in temporal focus are also easily found. Spanish-Americans, who have been described as taking the view that man is a victim of natural forces, are also a people who give a first order position to Present-Time. They pay little attention to what has happened in the past and regard the future as a vague and most unpredictable period. Planning for the future or hoping that the future will be better than either present or past simply is not their way of life.

Historic China was a society that gave first order value preference to Past-Time. Ancestor worship and a strong family tradition were both expressions of a Past-Time orientation. So also was the Chinese attitude that nothing new ever happened in the present or would happen in the future; it had all happened before in the far distant past.

Americans, more strongly than most peoples of the world, place an emphasis upon the future—a future that is anticipated as 'bigger and better'. This does not mean they have no regard for the past or thought of the present. But it certainly is true that no current generation of Americans ever wants to be called 'old-fashioned'. The ways of the past are not considered good just because they are past, and truly dominant Americans are seldom content with the present. This view results in a high evaluation of *change*, providing the change does not threaten the existing value order—the American way of life.

4. *Activity Orientation.* The modality of human activity is the fourth of the common human problems giving rise to a value-orientation system. The range of variation in solutions suggested for it is the three-fold one of Being, Being-in-Becoming, and Doing.

In the Being orientation the preference is for the kind of activity which is a spontaneous expression of what is conceived to be 'given' in the human personality. In some sense, this orientation is a spontaneous expression in activity of impulses and desires; yet care must be taken not to make this interpretation a too literal one. In no society, as Clyde Kluckhohn has commented, does one ever find a one-to-one relationship between the desired and the desirable. The *concrete behaviour of individuals in complex situations and the moral codes governing that behaviour usually reflect all the orientations simultaneously*. A stress upon the 'isness' of the personality and a spontaneous expression of that 'isness' is not pure licence, as we can easily see if we turn our attention to a society or segments of a society in which the Being orientation is the first order preference. Mexican society illustrates this preference well in its widely ramified patterning of *Fiesta* activities. Yet never in the *Fiesta*, with its emphasis on spontaneity, is there pure impulse gratification. The value demands of some of the other orientations made for codes which restrain the activities of the individuals in very definite ways.

The Being-in-Becoming orientation shares with the Being a great concern with what the human being is rather than what he can accomplish, but here the similarity ends. The idea of development, so little stressed in the Being orientation, is paramount in the Being-in-Becoming one. Erich Fromm's conception of 'the spontaneous activity of the total integrated personality' is close to but not identical with the Being-in-Becoming mode.

The Doing orientation is so characteristically the dominant one in American society that there is little need for an extensive discussion of it. Its most distinguishing feature is a demand for the kind of activity that results in accomplishment achieved by acting upon persons, things, or situations. What the individual does, and what he can or will accomplish, are almost always the primary questions in the American's scale of appraisal of persons. 'Getting things done' and 'Let's *do* something about it' are stock American phrases.

Fromm also considers this orientation to be different from the one he defines in his concept of spontaneity, but he does not accord it an equally favoured position. Instead he actually condemns it as a fertile source of neurotically compulsive behaviour. Although few would disagree that the Doing orientation of Americans makes for a competition with others which is often extreme and intense, it has not as yet been demonstrated that such competition customarily leads to or reflects compulsiveness in the technical sense of the term.

5. *Relational Orientation*. The last of the common human problems to be treated is the definition of man's relation to other men. This orientation has three subdivisions; the Lineal, the Collateral, and the Individualistic.

Individual autonomy is always found even in the most extreme types of *gemeinschaft* societies—that is, folk societies. The like-mindedness and behavioural similarities of individuals in 'homogeneous' groups have been overstressed. It is usually, if not always, the case that considerable leeway is permitted for individuality within the confines of the definitely fixed customs which *gemeinschaft* groups require for the ordering of human relationships. Individuality and individualism are both results of attention being given to the autonomy of the individual, but they are vastly different concepts, and significant nuances of meaning are lost when, as is so often the case, they are either confused or equated. There is actually less opportunity for a truly spontaneous individuality of expression in an individualistic society than in other, more fixed and firmly regulated, social orders. But, on the other hand, the man in an individualistic society need not remain in a fixed position and need not so often bow his head in acceptance of a dominating authority. He is much more 'free to be like everyone else.'

Collaterality also is found in all societies. The individual is not a human being except as he is a part of a social order, and one type of inevitable social grouping is that which results from laterally extended relationships. These are the more immediate relationships in time and space. Biologically, sibling relationships are the prototype of the Collateral relationship.

In addition, all societies must take into account the fact that individuals are biologically and culturally related to each other through time. There is, in other words, always a Lineal principle in relationships which is derived both from age and generational differences and from cultural continuity.

There will always be a variability, within systems and sub-systems as well as between them, in the primacy and the nature of goals which is in accord with variable stressing of the three principles. When the Individualistic principle is dominant, individual goals have primacy over the goals of specific Collateral or Lineal groups. This in no sense means that there is licence for the individual to pursue selfishly his own interests and in so doing disregard the interests of others. It is simply that each individual's responsibility to the total society and his place in it are in terms of goals (and roles) which are defined and structured as *autonomous* ones in the sense of being independent of particular Lineal or Collateral groupings.

A dominant Collateral orientation calls for a primacy of the goals and welfare of the laterally extended group. The group in this case is always moderately independent of other similar groups, and the problem of a well-regulated continuity of group relationships through time is not highly critical. The Navaho extended families and the loosely articulated combinations of these in what Clyde Kluckhohn calls an 'outfit' are illustrations of such groups. One also finds collaterality dominant in Italian culture. And although the individual Navaho or Italian always has some autonomous roles and some individualistic goals, and always also has some roles and goals that relate to a wider system viewed as continuous in time, the roles and goals that have primacy for him are those that are *representative* of his extended household group or 'outfit'.

If it is the Lineal principle that is dominant, it is again group goals that have primacy, but there is the additional factor that one of the most important of those group goals is continuity through time. *Continuity* of the group through time and ordered positional succession within the group are both crucial issues when Lineality dominates the relational system. Although other patterns are possible, it appears that the most successful means of maintaining a Lineal emphasis are either those based squarely upon hereditary factors such as primogeniture or those that are assimilated to a kinship structure.

To delineate the value-orientation profiles of the three groups included in the research monographs, histories, novels, and other sources were used. It is possible to test directly for the ranking of the orientations, but we have not as yet been able to do this for our sample.[1] These profiles are now given in Table 2, but given with the warning that 'ethnic labels' can be dangerous. For example, some Italians and some Irish-Americans, most certainly variants in their homeland, were more attuned to dominant American middle-class values at the time they arrived in this country than are many Old Yankees after several hundred years of participation in United States culture. But we need the modal (typical) orientation profiles as a base line for the analysis of the difference between the problems expected and those found. Therefore, in Table 2 the modal profiles of the dominant Middle-Class American, the Italian-American, and the Irish-American are drawn to the extent that we feel much certainty about them. For both the Italians and the Irish, the positions stated are those to which it is assumed a majority of the two groups held when they came to the United States.

As for the American middle-class case, I shall not take time to cite more than a few of the well-known facts. Parents are much concerned with the performance of their children, and training is ideally for in-

[1] In the research done on five sub-cultures in the American Southwest—Zuni, Navaho, Spanish-Americans, Mormons, and Texans—a research instrument was developed for a direct testing. The instrument and the results obtained with it appear in *Variations in Value Orientations*, op. cit.

Table 2 Culture

Orientation	Middle-Class American	Italian-American	Irish-American
Relational	Ind>Coll>Lin	Coll>Lin>Ind	Lin>Coll>Ind
Time	Fut>Pres>Past	Pres>Past>Fut	Pres>Past>Fut (but some indication of an earlier Past>Pres>Fut)
Man-Nature	Over>Subj>With	Subj>With>Over	Sub=With>Over (doubt about first order here and some doubt that there is a clear-cut first order preference)
Activity	Doing>Being>Being-in-Becoming	Being>Being-in-Becoming>Doing	Being>Being-in-Becoming>Doing
Human Nature	Evil>Mixed>Good Mixed Evil and Good>Evil>Good	Mixed Good and Evil predominantly	Most definitely an Evil basic nature with perfectibility desired but problematic

dependence of action and a show of initiative. Property gets classified as 'mine and thine'. Competitive behaviour is rewarded and success acclaimed. The child is also quite typically the hope of the future for many families, most especially those where parents have not themselves gone as far as they had hoped to go. The family is quite individualized, and relations with relatives of the extended family, either Lineal or Collateral, are not usually strong. Extended relations certainly are not held to if the holding is regarded as detrimental to the social mobility of the particular nuclear family.

Of all known families, this one is probably the best suited to our highly rationalized economic system and other spheres of our national life. It does produce achievement-minded, independent, and future-oriented individuals who are largely free of ties that bind them in time and place. Critics of the American family all too often forget to consider the wider social system and the meshing of family and other institutions.

But the critics are correct in pointing to the numerous strains on individuals which are more or less endemic in such a family. There are many strains on women as wives and mothers, on men as husbands and fathers, and these, separately and in relation to each other, inevitably have effects upon developing children. Much has been written on all the strains and their effects. Erik Erikson, for one, has provided us with a most penetrating analysis in the chapter on 'The American Identity' in his *Childhood and Society*.[1] Many books and articles have been devoted to the analysis of the American feminine role, to the American mother-child relationship, and some even to the roles men play as husbands and fathers.

In illustrating our use of the value-orientation theory for a diagnosis and interpretation of family relations, I shall first discuss some aspects of the Italian patterns. If one turns back to the table that lists the orientations of all three cultures, it is easily noted that there is a wide range difference between the value preferences of the typical Italian and the middle-class American on all orientations. In each case, if the Italian is to become a thorough-going middle-class American in his basic values, he must move from his own first order preferences to what has been in the past his third order and least favoured value choices. This is no easy move for any people to make and certainly not one that can be made quickly without creating problems. It has long been my contention that the assimilation process for peoples coming into this country will vary in accord with the degree of goodness of fit between the value orientations they brought with them and the dominant values of the society. When people have markedly different value preferences on all the orientations, the process will be slower and more fraught with difficulties than if there were agreement on some one or two. And the most difficult change of all is the radical shift to value positions that formerly had been the least favoured of all.

All the Italian families of our sample are in process of movement away from typical Italian values to those of the dominant culture, but there are differences in both rate and kind of movement between the 'sick' and 'well' families. The most critical difference seems to be the order of change by orientation. In the 'sick' families there has been, for one reason or another, a breakdown of the Collateral *relational* ties, whereas in the well families these ties are still quite strong. It is one thing to try to change from a non-planning Present-Time and Being oriented position when one has the 'cushion' of ramified family ties to support and sustain one in case of failures, but quite another thing when these are lacking. The pacing of change and the cognitive grasp of the difference between goals and the means of attaining them and the relation of means to goals are the other striking criteria by which the two kinds of families can be differentiated.

In the Italian families defined as 'sick' the Collateral ties have been partially or wholly destroyed, and there is not as yet in any of them a

[1] Erik H. Erikson, *Childhood and Society*, W. W. Norton & Co., New York, 1950.

sufficient understanding of an Individualistic relational orientation for them to operate successfully as 'isolated nuclear' families. They are stranded and confused; virtually in a void as far as relations with others are concerned. They also all show small ability to instrument their plans and desires for the material things or other of the goals of middle-class culture which they have come to consider important goals. The well families, in contrast, have maintained quite good Collateral ties on both sides of the family—and relative both to goals set and the means of attaining them, they are far more 'realistic'.

All these families have problems, many of them very similar in origin, in nature, and in degree. It is the handling of them which varies so greatly. In the well families there is, in addition to the more realistic grasp of the relation of means to ends, a greater ability on the part of the parents to look problems in the face and communicate with each other about them. The parents in the sick families have poor communication with each other, and they characteristically deny that there are tensions between them or that they are in any way to blame for the problems they face. They project onto the outside world, but more important still they also have found a focus for projection within the family itself—a particular child.

Let me illustrate briefly from two cases. In one—one where we have had little success in the treatment of the family—the father and mother have both had troubles with their extended families, and they feel that in no way can they count on the relatives to help them out; they also, partly because of these same relatives, are a 'looked down upon' family in the community (largely Italian) in which they live. There is a great deal of friction between themselves which scarcely ever comes out into the open. In fact one of the main reasons for the failure of therapy in this family was that, every time the therapist of the father or the mother came close to bringing to the fore the problems between them, there was a withdrawal on the part of one or both. The father in particular was extremely reluctant to co-operate if co-operation meant any discussion of himself or his relationships.

Teachers of their children, the doctors whom they sought out in great variety, employers, and neighbours whom they accused of spying upon them were frequent targets for their feelings of failure and frustration. But it was their first child, a little girl of ten years with a low level of intelligence who was the main target for the projection of their problems. They constantly assigned to this child the implicit and informal roles of 'the bad girl', 'the girl who was and would always be a disgrace to them', 'the child who was a cross to bear'. The child is, indeed, a difficult case. Not only is her intelligence low, but she is the closest to being an atypical child of any that we had in our sample. But one may, and we did, question how much of her most bizarre behaviour and her lack of ability to perform in school were effects of the roles that both the father and mother have assigned to her. Certainly it is a fact that the parents have been (1) strongly resistant to facing the possibility that the main problems are in themselves rather than in this one child and (2) almost equally resistant to agreeing to anything that might really help the child. In other words, her aberrant behaviour, which they certainly in some part induce, seems to be necessary for the maintenance of what family equilibrium does exist.

In another case, not dissimilar in general outline, we were more successful in treatment but only after a very long period of time. This family, too, was cut off from ties with the extended families of both father and mother, and there was an even greater feeling of isolation relative to the community in which they lived. Here the child singled out as a problem child upon whom many kinds of frustrations and anxieties could be projected was a little girl, the second of the family, who again was less bright than her siblings. But another factor in the focusing of attention upon this particular child was that after a long siege of rheumatic fever that she had had, her doctors, all middle-class Americans, had insisted that special attention be accorded her. She was to have a room to herself, a special kind of bed, and other attentions that did not fit in at all well with the Collateral patterning of Italian families. This special treatment increased resentment towards her and made her the better target for all kinds of tensions. And here again the informal and implicit roles assigned to her were that she was untrustworthy, irresponsible, and would always be a probable source of disgrace to the family in the wider community. The additional one was that she was demanding in a way 'good' Italian children should not be.

Obviously, in these and all our other cases, the factor of value conflict is only one of many to be considered. But its importance becomes most apparent when one compares families that are so very similar in many ways but very different in the degree to which acculturation is a problem for family equilibrium.

The significance of the value factor is made even more obvious when the acculturation processes of different groups are compared. In the Irish-American group, for example, one finds different problems because the shifts in value positions which the Irish have had to make, if and when they become assimilated, are different from those Italians must make.

But rather than give the details of this comparison, I wish to illustrate from the Irish-American case another use of the value-orientation theory in the analysis of family problems. This use is the prediction of the kinds of strains one is likely to find common in a system because of the particular combination of basic values adhered to in a culture and the further strains that are produced when acculturation occurs.

In our analysis of the culture of rural Irish we were especially struck by the possibilities for much *intra-cultural* strain because of the juxtaposition in the total value system of a very strong first order Lineal *relational* orientation[1] and a dominant human-nature orientation which is a more extreme version of the Evil but perfectible position than even that adhered to by New England Puritans. This particular combination of value orientations requires on the one hand a training of persons for dependent behaviour and a low degree of individual responsibility, but on the other keeps them ever conscious of an evil nature which they *themselves* must control. The Yankee Puritan whose dominant *relational* orientation was Individualism was not caught in this dilemma of contradictions. Thus, we expected to find, fairly typically, in the Irish group strong denial and escape mechanisms. More concretely, we predicted that members of the group would commonly deny responsibility for happenings, including consequences of their acts, but that they also would have intense guilt feelings. It was further predicted that escape patterns would be prevalent—most especially in cases where men in their occupational roles had been thrown too much and too soon into situations demanding much individual responsibility and quite independent action. Conversely, it was expected that there would be fewer instances of either of these defence mechanisms in cases where men had found employment in organizations, governmental or otherwise, which were quite Lineal in character. It was also expected that sexuality would be a source of great anxiety to this group.

On the whole our findings have accorded well with our expectations. The prevalence of the denial and escape defence mechanisms has been striking indeed. Treatment of the 'sick' Irish-American families has been greatly handicapped because issues and problems are so often and so strongly denied. Moreover, it has been our experience that it is difficult to keep Irish-American families in treatment.

These few illustrations must serve to indicate how we have found the factor of basic values—value orientations—critical to the analysis of family relations.

[1] The best *single* source of information on the Lineal *relational* structure of modern rural Ireland is: Conrad M. Arensberg and Solon T. Kimball, *Family and Community in Ireland*, Harvard University Press, Cambridge, 1940.

6

ARE WE CREATING DEPENDENCY?*

HELEN HARRIS PERLMAN

DEPENDENCY is a bad word. It has done some loose living on the tongues of many people; it has kept questionable company with other bad words like 'pauperization' and 'welfare state'; it has been under attack by a group of highly respectable myths; and it has a way of making some people angry and other people uneasy. So it is most understandable that social workers feel some anxiety when they are accused of being instrumental in creating this bad thing.

The professional social worker has been trained to attempt to understand the exact nature of a problem before trying to deal with it. Therefore, I am impelled to take this bad word out into the light and see, first of all, what it is and what it means, and then I should like to separate it from some of the dubious company it keeps and from the myths which deplore it. Only then can we answer the question: Are we creating dependency? Then I should like to add to it another question: Can social workers do anything to prevent it?

Dependency has been defined as 'the state of being at the disposal of another, sustained by another, relying upon another's support or favour'. To be dependent is to be unable to exist or sustain one's self or perform anything without the will power or aid of something or someone else.

Immediately we come face to face with a ubiquitous myth. This myth enters alternately slapping his chest and tugging at his boot straps. He announces in a loud voice that he is an independent man, self-made; nobody gives him anything, and he owes nothing to anyone. You will detect a hollow sound as he beats his chest, however, and if he hears but one voice of disbelief he will vanish into thin air. This is because there is no real independent man, unless he is a self-appointed hermit on a desert island. Every normal human being in our society is dependent

* Published in *The Social Service Review*, Vol. XXXIV, No. 3, September, 1960. This article originally appeared in the June, 1951 issue of *Minnesota Welfare*.

in a number of areas of his living. We are dependent on other persons for their love, their esteem, their great or small kindnesses. We are dependent on the occupational functions of other people, on other persons' maintaining certain circumstances necessary for our well-being, on other persons' production and consumption. According to our age, capacities, personal resources, and life-circumstances, our dependency upon other persons and other things will vary in depth and scope. Total self-dependence is an illusion in today's interlaced society. The necessity to give and take, to nurture and to feed upon, to carry certain responsibilities and to expect certain rights—these make up the normal balance between dependency and independence. This balance in the adult person can be called *relative* self-dependence.

Another confusion about this word 'dependency' needs to be examined. In newspaper articles, in legislators' thinking, in political speeches, even in social workers' communications with one another, there has been a tendency to pair economic dependency with psychological dependency, that is, to speak as if the individual's need to take financial support automatically placed him in the position of needing to lean on others for support in other areas of his living. Thus people who are economically dependent on public assistance are assumed to be less self-reliant, more lazy, less responsible, more weak, simply by virtue of their need for money which they do not earn. These assumptions need careful examination.

Economic dependency may be said to be a condition of having to rely upon some source of income which the individual does not earn by his labours or endeavours. Psychological dependency is a state of having to rely upon some human being's power, nurture, initiative outside one's self because of one's feeling of insecurity and helplessness. Obviously, all people, economically self-dependent though they may be, have moments or periods or psychological dependency, and some people who are economically self-dependent may be chronically dependent psychologically. It is also true that economic and psychological dependency may occur together. Either one may be the cause of the other, but they may be found each without the other, and the existence of one does not automatically bespeak the existence of the other. Thus a man taking relief for reasons of physical disability may fully retain his capacities as a husband or father, a club member, a citizen—may operate, in short, like a self-dependent person except in the area of his ability to earn. On the other hand, a man with what we call, interestingly enough, an 'independent income' may be bankrupt as far as productive use of himself is concerned, may be a useless parasite.

We are confronted by a second myth which beclouds our thinking when we speak of 'relief' and 'dependency' as if they were inevitably linked. This myth obviously comes from a long line of eminently respectable myths. You can tell this by the silver buckles on his shoes and the slightly frayed lace at his cuffs and by the way he looks down his thin, tight nose. Despite the fact that he is hopelessly superannuated and has good reason to be dead, he continues to haunt the premises of old people's minds by asserting that only shiftless and immoral persons are poor—or, at least only these stay poor. Most of the people of this century in this country know that this is nonsense—yet so insidiously respectable is this myth that he is allowed living room in people's thinking, and they find themselves unwittingly believing in him and being victimized by him. We come out, somehow, tacitly accepting that virtue and vice are economic class attributes. As an example: depending on our particular sympathies, we flinch or we are indignant when a 'chiseler' is found on the relief rolls. Is it not naive of us to expect that all the poor are or can be expected to be honest? Do we make such blanket expectation of people in other income brackets? Obviously not. Chiselers are found in economically self-dependent groups, too—income tax chiselers, for example. And our reaction to those chiselers, too, is that they have been dishonest. But is it not interesting that no public voice says that men who make over $10,000 a year are all tax dodgers and that lack of moral stamina is an inevitable accompaniment to economic well-being? Yet generalizations equally ludicrous are made about all the people who are poor enough to need economic assistance. They are on relief; therefore, says the myth, whether they be young or old, Protestant or Catholic, male or female, sick or well, bright or dull, in chronic or temporary need, labourers or white-collar workers, all of them, says the myth, are alike—they are all people who are lacking in moral stamina.

The most troubling part of the influence of this myth is that the accusation of psychological dependency is levelled at the economically dependent as a way of degrading and shaming them, as a way of saying 'they wouldn't be poor if they were any good'. And because the economically dependent person is not a man apart, because he reads the newspaper and hears the accusations on tongues about him and per-haps even sees that accusation in the eyes of his social worker, he begins himself to believe it. He begins to feel like something less than a worth-while person, like something of a second-class citizen, and respect for himself begins to crumble. Psychological dependency may begin with such loss of self-respect.

As for the social worker, the necessity for his taking a good look at words and myths is not just a precious exercise in semantics. It is of considerable importance in answering just such a question as we face today. Firstly, he must recognize that, despite all rumours to the contrary, the social worker does not create the situations which make for human dependency. Then, in order to answer whether he is creating psychological dependency, he must ask: How does psychological dependency come about? What is its relation, if any, to social work programmes and practices?

The push and thrust of the human body and spirit for self-dependence may be said to be born in us. It is present from birth in greater or lesser degree in every individual. Perhaps its comparative strength or weakness has something to do with inheritance or constitutional structure—nobody really knows. One baby sits like a placid Buddha and broods at the world and another dances out of its skin; but every healthy baby shows from its early days an impulse to do on its own in spite of the fact that its dependency needs are being met by loving, cradling parents. Every baby begins to kick and bounce, to grasp, to say, by its actions, 'I do not simply sit and wait for you—I want, I will get, I will do for myself.' He pulls himself up on the side of his crib, he crawls after a plaything, he mashes his hand into his oatmeal and pushes it into his face, he begins to venture about in the jungle of tables and chair legs, he experiments with the sound of crashing pots and pans, and often, when his parents try to put some limits on his exercise of self-dependence, he screams in protest at their effort to make him subject to their will.

Now, in the average family, along with the baby's own natural development, certain achievements are set up for his attainment, that is, certain expectations are held for him. He is expected to begin to use feeding utensils, to control his impulses to swat the cat or grab toys from a playmate. He begins to be trained to be both self-dependent and interdependent, to exercise his rights, and to take the concomitant responsibilities. These expectations of him will continue, although their forms will change. As he grows he will be expected to leave the protection of his mother and go off to school, to begin to study, to carry some tasks, to learn to use money, to plan in advance, to make decisions, to strive to achieve some place for himself as student or worker and, eventually, as key member of a new family. When he comes to maturity he will be, it is hoped, a person able and willing to carry his share of the load, able and willing to be a dependable member of an independent society.

But all this does not just happen. Certain conditions must be provided to make it happen. The basic conditions to growth in the baby, in the child, and in the adult are compounded of three ingredients: firstly, that feeling of safety, that knowledge of basic support which is called security; secondly, the presence of tangible material resources to use in play and work; and, thirdly, the knowledge that there is some reward for taking a risk, for trying—the reward of being loved or of being gratified. This is what gives the child and the adult free energy to reach out beyond himself for new learning and growth. The young child's security lies in knowing that home and family are a place where he is wanted and loved, that school is a place where people help him learn many things, that three meals and clean jeans and a pair of roller skates may be taken for granted; and when this security is had, the child is ready to reach out for new experiences. The adolescent's security lies in knowing that he is not a bad-looking fellow, and that he is respected by his schoolmates and his teachers, and that his parents, though they may argue with him, really stand behind him, that they will strive to provide him with opportunity to try his wings, and that his efforts to study or work will be fruitful. As we grow older we are secured not simply by what we have today, but we begin to have foresight and the need to have some feeling of security ahead of us. So the maturing adolescent needs to know that his efforts and his ambitions will yield him some rewards. When he has these securities he feels strong, and he is able to give himself over to developing his abilities and using his opportunities. In other words, in the average human being, growth, initiative, and self-dependence require a floor of security from which to build.

What, then, has happened to those persons who come to adulthood with feelings of insecurity, of inadequacy and fearfulness, who, whether they are economically dependent or not, are considered to be irresponsible or neurotic or dependent? What happened to their natural endowment of energy pushing out for self-realization and self-dependence? Probably something like this: Through the childhood and young adulthood of these persons the floor of security was missing—or, at least, was full of dangerous holes. Through their development they found evidence that theirs was a world to make one more fearful than confident. They experienced more hurt than comfort, they felt more deprivation than fulfilment. Deprivation and frustration can be of many sorts. They may take the form of consistently harsh parents who demand more of the child than they give him, who make more of his failures than of his successes, who, in short, fill him with the sense that 'it's no use trying because I'm not much good'. This kind of deprivation may occur in any social class, and among the rich as well as the poor one may find the individual whose life-energy is bound up alternately in despising himself and licking his wounds, and in hating those who hurt him. When we find this individual in the economically independent group, he is called a 'neurotic' or is said to have an 'inferiority complex'. When we find him in the economically deprived group, we tend to say he is 'shiftless', 'pauperized', 'dependent'.

Another source of an individual's helplessness and irresponsibility may be those parents who unwittingly rob the growing child of his rights to self-dependence by carrying all the responsibility for him, binding him hand and foot, as it were. Though their cords may be silken they are incapacitating to his self-dependence and initiative. The adult product of this form of deprivation will be found in all economic classes, too. When he is found among the rich he is seen, sometimes indulgently, sometimes censoriously, as a playboy or a mamma's boy or a parasite. When he is found on the relief rolls he may be a 'good client', an obedient one, but he lacks 'get up', and he may look to the caseworker to tell him what to do and how to do it; he is called 'pauperized' and 'dependent'.

Yet a third group of factors may make for psychological dependence. These are experiences or circumstances an individual encounters that attack him so shockingly and overwhelmingly, are so deeply disappointing, that he retreats from the struggle with them and seeks safety. Safety may be found at some earlier level of adjustment where he felt less attacked, or it may be found in reliance upon something outside himself. In the economically secure individual the momentary cataclysm or the chronic derangement of his life-situation may be cushioned by money. It can buy him escape or substitute ways of seeking satisfactions, and his helplessness is mitigated somewhat. But for the person who has no cushioning, whose weakness is only emphasized by his being economically dependent, the sense of insecurity and hopelessness is likely to be heavy. Unless he experiences some relationship and/or some situation in which he can feel safe again, in which he can see a ray of hope and can risk taking another chance on himself, he is likely to resign himself to depending on what seems safe for survival, inadequate though it may be.

The signs by which one can detect psychological dependency are not that the individual gets aid to dependent children, old age assistance, or general assistance. They are, rather, the presence of feelings of resignation, helplessness, hostile pessimism, physical sickness for which doctors can find no organic base, passivity, and inability to mobilize the self to take necessary action or responsibilities.

Every practising social worker can testify that the necessity to take financial help does not in itself create psychological dependency. The A.D.C.[1] worker knows large numbers of mothers. They keep their homes and their children clean, they cook the proper foods, they send their children to school, they comfort them when they are sick, and take pleasure in them when they do well, they train them in acceptable habits and behaviour—in short, they fulfil all the duties and carry all the responsibilities of normal motherhood. The worker with the blind knows large numbers of the sightless who maintain steady family and community relationships, who work at learning to occupy themselves constructively, who emphasize their capacities rather than their disabilities, who, in short, lead their own lives as responsibly as it is possible to do within their darkened world. The O.A.A.[2] worker knows numerous men and women who cook, sew and care for themselves, who seek friendships and lend a frail but helping hand to neighbours, who, as statistics of the World War II period showed, literally rushed to remunerative work when it was open to them, who, in short, carry out all the normal obligations of the aged in our society. The general assistance worker knows men and women who, despite the calamity which has resulted in their economic dependency, maintain good strong family life, go to church, vote, school their children, and hope and plan for the day when they or at least their children will be on their own feet again. (Incidentally in a long and broad social work experience, I have never known one person, not one, who looked forward to his child's growing up and getting 'on relief'.) All these people are psychologically self-dependent, responsible persons. They are sound citizens with empty purses.

Some persons receiving assistance are both economically and psychologically dependent. The proportion or number of these has not been established by anyone. It is a peculiar phenomenon that when one such person appears he is sometimes seen as if he were twins or quadruplets or, by that odd distortion of vision that bias creates, he is seen multiplied by the hundreds. However that may be, there are individuals—number unknown—on relief loads who are not self-responsible persons, who depend on others to do for them. Such persons are our concern, both as social workers and as citizens in a democracy. Our

[1] Aid to Dependent Children.
[2] Old Age Assistance.

concern is that it should not be the social welfare programme or the methods caseworkers use which drain them of their self-sufficiency.

Every one of us knows that in order to be adequate to the day's work one must feel physically adequate. A headache can immobilize a person, a toothache can put all the feeling and thinking into one small cavity. When one is hungry, one's mind is split between the task at hand and the demands of the stomach. In all of the common experiences of the human body we know how closely tied together are our feelings of physical well-being and our feeling of ability to cope with our small or big daily programme.

Most of the men and women and children receiving public assistance today are chronically underfed or poorly fed. The so-called marginal food budget on which families on relief live is in the face of present food prices actually submarginal. As a woman who buys and plans family meals, I know the daily shock of seeing the chain store cash register leap to add up dollars for basic necessities of food, and there is no day when I do not wonder how mothers on A.D.C. manage to feed their children well enough so that they have energy to play and work at school. Many of them cannot, of course, and they and the old and the handicapped, and those for whom no category of relief has yet been established, live day after day, month after month, poorly, monotonously, and underfed. Their physical energy is bound to be low. Their psychic energy is likewise sapped. The 'get-up', the 'go-after', the vitality, the planfulness—all those attributes which are the concomitants of self-dependence—are, just like the budget, likely to be marginal rather than adequate. But, more than this, the marginal living standard has its constant psychic component. It presents continuous evidence that the world is a mean place to live in.

Under these circumstances what is likely to happen to the person? Is he likely to feel hopeful, optimistic? Is he likely to feel gratified and adequate to deal with his daily problems? It would be unusual if this happened. He is more likely to feel resentful or hostile, chronically unsatisfied—or to take on the characteristics attributed to him and feel ashamed and resigned and needful. These are the characteristics of dependency. It is this experience of exhausting, pinching, and chronic economic deprivation of the barely adequate relief grant which can contribute heavily to feelings of psychological dependency.

At this point a pair of myths inevitably arise to confront us, and we must take cognizance of them. One of them wears his head backwards on his shoulders. He is rapt in his admiration of the past. 'In those days,' he will tell you, 'there were giants. In those days men dragged the stones that built their houses, they pushed or pulled their ploughs; women carried water and boiled soap and brewed medicine; children went barefooted and were glad to eat what they got. People would have died rather than ask for help—they were giants.' This myth does not realize, of course, that only the giants had loud enough voices to tell their tales. The voices of those who sickened and warped and died before their time were quiet voices that could be heard only by those who cared to hear them. This myth's twin brother has eyes and ears stretched out of shape by focusing on far horizons. 'In some countries,' he will tell you, 'people are satisfied with bread and cheese'.

It is interesting that while both these myths are as thin as air they are not readily dispelled. What must be said to exorcise them is that 'in those times' is not now, and 'in that place', is not here. We are living, and so are persons on relief, here and now, in the second half of the twentieth century, in the United States of America. Materialistic values are high. One may decry this, but it is a fact. The things one must eat to be well, wear to be accepted, own to 'belong', are infinitely multiplied over what they were even fifty years ago. Moreover, it is a time when knowledge of what people have a right to want is spread by unending communication from radios, newspapers, billboards, movies. Only recently the chairman of one of America's greatest corporations said, 'There is a definite correlation between education and the consumption of commodities.' Had he been speaking of persons on relief he might have added, 'or in the sense of need for those commodities'.

Every person's sense of his needs is greater, far greater, than was the sense of need of fifty years ago. My grandfather said that he never saw an orange until he was twelve years old, and when he ate it, rind and all, he wondered why people considered it such a delicacy. Nowadays every mother considers oranges a basic need for her baby's health. People's felt needs rise and multiply as standards of living rise and become more complex. It is fallacious to speak of the days when one's grandfather raised seven fine sons in a one-room log cabin, because this took place in a different setting, a different time, a different culture from ours today. In a culture of one-room log cabins the seven sons grew up feeling equal to their peers. In a culture in which people are supposed to have bedrooms, the sense of inequality is keen when these cannot be had. In a community where bread and cheese are the normal diet, people will live on bread and cheese with equanimity, even though the sickness rate among them may be appalling. In a community where people know that balanced diets secure health and where, moreover, lavish varieties of foods spill over from grocery counters and coloured advertisements, the person who must confine himself to bread and cheese feels both cheated and defeated.

The fact is that at our present stage of technological and psychological development nobody considers subsistence living to be enough to meet his needs. Sometimes we consider it to be enough for somebody else, but never for ourselves. Nor does the client on relief consider it to be enough for himself. He may feel it is all he deserves, or know it is all he can hope for. But underneath seethes the feeling that there is a very great disparity between what he wants or thinks he needs and what his society gives him. He is left with a sense of being a second-class member of the community; feelings of frustration and helplessness may undermine the sense of adequacy and security which is basic to his self-dependence.

We said before that a potent factor in creating or abetting psychological dependency is that of hopelessness, of feeling that there is no way out, nothing better to look forward to. This robs people of all incentive. Yet, unwittingly, hopelessness seems almost written into some relief programmes. When youngsters must leave school, not because they have fulfilled their capacities and educational interests, but because they are old enough to earn money to supplement the family's relief grant, when a man's or woman's effort to do some work brings only a threat of being cut off from relief before he has adequately tested the job or his capacity to carry it, when a man discharged from a tuberculosis sanatorium returns to the same skimpy diet and dingy rooms that first helped to inflame his lungs, when adolescents find that out of their newly won earnings they must turn over to the family everything but the cost of working, when a man found in the home of an A.D.C. mother is viewed either as an undesirable source of income or sin, when, in short, the hopes of bettering one's self, of having things different, are consistently cut off, then hope flies out the window and with it the spirit that makes people want to continue to struggle for self-realization and self-dependence.

Since a programme of economic assistance is only a subsistence programme, the individual will subsist, that is, he will exist marginally. His energies will be enough for survival and he will have little surplus. When a person lives at this marginal level for long periods of time with nothing to hope for, there will develop in him a sense of ill-being, of emptiness, of needfulness and hopelessness. These are the very essence of psychological dependency.

Therefore the adequacy or inadequacy of a welfare programme—its mean or decent meeting of basic human needs—will have a potent influence in creating, abetting, or preventing psychological dependency.

Now we must turn to the social workers themselves, those who administer and convey the assistance agency's service. Do they, by the way they feel and act and deal with people, create or encourage dependency? Or do they have means for the modification or prevention of dependency?

Social caseworkers may be tremendously important persons in the lives of the people they touch. This is because the client experiences the social agency largely through his individual social worker. For the average client, his worker's attitude represents the agency's attitude towards him and, back of that, the community's attitude towards him. As agency representative to the client, and as interpreter of client to the agency, the social worker is in a vital position to affect the lives of the people the agency helps.

By the way the social caseworker relates himself to and deals with him, his client's sense of personal worth may be enhanced. By the adequacy and dependability of the agency's helping services, the floor of security may be steadied. By the provisions of community resources outside the agency and the stimulus to the use of those resources, that sense of possible fulfilment, which is hope, may be buoyed.

In the run of everyday practice what does this involve? Everyone of us wants and needs the respect of other people—in a sense we live by the image of ourselves which we see reflected in the eyes of another. The more important that other person is to us—the more he represents established values—the more we want to be accepted by him. When he accepts us and shows his respect for us, we are strengthened in our convictions about our self-worth. That is true of our clients, too. The social caseworker represents the agency and the community, and because of this he is more than just himself to the client. The evidence he gives that he respects the client, that he is sincerely interested in him, that he appreciates his difficulties, that he assumes and affirms that the client has the full rights and responsibilities of a first-class citizen—this evidence strengthens the client's wish to operate as a first-class citizen.

Sometimes, either because of our own emotions or because of our lack of understanding, we tend to deal with the client as if we thought that economic and psychological dependency were the same thing. When this happens, we may be impatient, punishing, and overauthoritative or, conversely, overprotective, as if to imply 'We consider you a bad child' or 'You are a poor thing.' The client senses this implication. He may react in various ways, but the end result is that he feels like a 'bad child' or a 'poor thing' and thereby his sense of self-worth is lessened. This has implications for what we do together with our client as well as how we act towards him. In the everyday interview with the everyday client some problem of his current living is discussed: How can I manage on my budget? How can I get my husband to meet his court order? What shall I do about my toothaches? What shall I do about my child's hating school? If we assume that he is psychologically dependent just because he is a client, if we assume that he is too dumb or too weak to think or do on his own, we may tend to think or do for him. The authoritative worker says, 'Sign this, do that, go there, and for goodness' sake get going.' The over-protective caseworker says, 'I'll figure that out, I'll tell you what to do, I'll do it for you.' In the first instance the client is robbed of his rights, in the second he is robbed of his responsibility; either robs him of the exercise of his self-dependence.

But the caseworker who understands the nature of self-dependence knows that it grows on help to use one's own powers. Therefore the caseworker offers help to his client in these ways: (1) He relates to him with compassion and understanding. (2) He stimulates him to think about ways and means of solving his problem, the possible action that he may take, the possible consequences of such action. (3) He makes known to the client the resources or means available to him. (4) He encourages him to consider what resources or means he may have in himself or his normal environment that can be used. (5) He helps him to come to some decision on his own as to what is the best thing to do. (6) He supports him in taking the next step by the demonstration and the assurance of the agency's standing by to give him help in case he fails. By these means of engaging the client's active thought and muscle in working on the particular day's problem, we exercise his strengths and help him to know and use his own capacities. The dependent person begins to feel the pleasure of the emerging powers in himself; the self-dependent person has his strengths tried and confirmed.

To feel respected and to feel able to cope with the small problems of everyday living are basic human needs. To these must be added something that will enable a person to lift up his eyes from today and look ahead to tomorrow—some motivation to keep going. Hope—or the reaching out for something beyond today—must be founded on something real. To say that anyone can be anything he chooses to be, do anything he is ambitious to do, is simply not true. I assume that social workers need hardly be told of the vast inequality of capacities with which individuals come into the world and the vast inequality of opportunity which they encounter here. This is one of the reasons for the existence of social work: that it should create or make attainable opportunities of which large numbers of people would otherwise be deprived. And this is why it is incumbent upon the social caseworker to do two things: first, to comb his community for those resources of medical, occupational, religious, recreational, educational opportunity and to help his clients know them and use them to enrich their lives; and, second, to make known to his own agency, to the churches, to the school, to men's and women's clubs, what resources need to be developed in order that the emptiness in people's lives may be filled. The blind man may not hope for sight again, or the aged for youth again, the disabled may not be well again, or the fatherless children have a normal home. But each of these may be helped to look beyond his immediate frustrations, may come to feel less helpless if the social caseworker can provide an injection of that hope which rises out of such commonplace opportunities as having a radio, going to a church social, getting materials for reading or handiwork, getting a set of teeth, garden seed, or a chance to go on a vacation. These opportunities empower people; they build up their morale, their feeling that life holds some interests and some satisfactions. Interest and some experience of satisfaction beyond keeping body and soul together— these are the bootstraps by which every one of us pulls himself up. Our clients need them too for the development of their self-dependence.

If social workers operate in these ways—by an understanding, respectful relationship to their clients, by helping them to recognize and exercise their own abilities to plan and work on their daily problems, by providing opportunities for the expanding use of themselves and for the hopefulness this excites—then social workers may be said to be ameliorating and even preventing dependency.

But the social worker too must be enabled. He must have the means and conditions of work that will permit him to consider and to do these things. When case loads are too high, for example, sustained contact with clients becomes impossible and only 'hit-and-run' visits can be made. Under those circumstances there is little chance that the client will come to relate to his caseworker, or trust him, or find him a source of helpfulness. Nor can the caseworker himself, under such conditions, do anything more than meet minimum requirements of investigation of need and provision of means. Like the Red Queen he must 'do all the running he can do to keep in the same place'. When salaries are too low, the exhausting and demanding business of dealing with troubled people provides little economic reward or security for the caseworker himself. Then staff turnover and unattended case loads will be inevitable. The too high case load and the too low salary are only two of the many administrative factors in today's public assistance agency which affect its workers' capacity to prevent or adequately to deal with psychological dependency when it is detected. Such factors ought not to be the concern of the social worker alone; they are the rightful concern of every citizen who fears the psychological effects of deprivation and hopelessness.

A critic of social work once proposed that social workers ought to stand, not for a 'Welfare State', but for an 'Incentive State'. 'Incentive' means rousing to action, encouraging, moving. To keep people active on their own behalf, to encourage them to move forward—these are the very tenets of social casework. From an understanding of the conditions which paralyse or motivate people, it would be hard to see how fear and want could generate incentive. If that were possible, our most enterprising and productive population would be the ill-fed, ill-housed and ill-clothed. And, conversely, our economically secure population would be intellectual and moral sluggards.

Social workers know that incentive, like self-dependence, is compounded of many things. It is made up of wish for status in the eyes of one's fellow men; of the wish to occupy one's self with something that is rewarding and satisfying; of the wish for more of the good things of living than relief payments or insurance benefits will ever buy; and of the desire to be something better than what one is today. We know, too, that in order for incentive, like self-dependence, to be sustained it must be underpinned by physical and mental well-being, by basic security, by open opportunity, and by some realistic grounds for looking forward with hope. It is those conditions that make for basic human welfare, for reasonable self-dependence, and for incentive that social workers must work for and help create.

7

CASEWORK AND AGENCY FUNCTION*

CLARE WINNICOTT

FOR a long time now I have wanted to try to explore further the question of agency function and its effect on the casework process. The subject has intrigued me. It is a very vital subject, and at the same time a practical one in view of the fact that caseworkers function within agencies. It seems to me especially important that as we move away from specialization both in training and in our professional life, we should try to understand more fully than ever the essential nature of the functions of each agency and the effect that these have on the case-workers who give them meaning for the client.

Recently in the Younghusband Report[1] (Chapter 12) we have had convincingly put before us evidence which shows that one factor con-tributing to the lack of co-ordination of the social services is the social worker's lack of clarity about the functions of other social services, and the lack of clarity about his or her own functions within a particular service. The Ingleby Committee[2] summarized and endorsed these findings.

The problem of defining functions within a social service and between the social services is, of course, one which must be tackled at all levels throughout the services, and must be seen from many different points of view. There is no doubt that only by effective co-operation can we make full use of the social provisions which we have been fortunate enough to achieve in this country. But as the Younghusband Report reminds us, the basis of co-operation is each one's confidence in his or her own function.

In what I shall say about casework and agency function I shall be focusing on one bit of this complex problem of defining functions, in

---

* Published in *Case Conference*, Vol. VIII, No. 7, January, 1962.
[1] *Report of the Working Party on Social Workers in the Local Authority Health and Welfare Services*, H.M.S.O., London, 1959.
[2] *Report of the Committee on Children and Young Persons*, H.M.S.O., London, 1960.

my view a vital bit, because it concerns the integration of casework function and agency function. I shall try to state the dynamics of agency function in casework terms.

Surprisingly enough this problem was seen as long ago as 1903 by Professor Urwick; he refreshingly stated, speaking of the practitioner of social work, that 'his methods must be made scientific, his practice must be founded on a true knowledge of principles of law; and he, the practitioner, must himself acquire that knowledge and be trained in these methods'. He goes on to say (and this is the important part) '(The social worker) must learn to realize the slow growth that lies behind each condition and fact; to see in the social structure whole or part, of state, or of institution, the expression of a vital meaning; to feel beneath the seemingly plastic relationships of social life, the framework of economic necessities; and to find in each causal tendency and habit the effect of slowly changing mental processes. Not the training of the man of science, but the scientific attitude, must be his; that at least is necessary if experience is to be used aright.'[1]

It is inspired creative thinking such as this that has led to our emergence as a profession. More recently we have been profoundly influenced in our development by the writings of American social workers who were able to see more quickly than we were that, in particular, the findings of dynamic psychology could and must be applied to social work if it were to move forward towards a greater understanding of individual social maladjustment. The work done by our American colleagues in refining out social work concepts from the application of theory to practice has given us the basic requirement of a profession, that is, a language in which to communicate essential ideas, and this we have taken over from them. We shall Anglicize it and alter it in the light of our own thinking and experience, but without it we should have had to start from scratch.

During recent years social caseworkers in all fields have been especially concerned with establishing themselves as a group of people bound together by common professional aims, standards, techniques and attitudes, a group whose entity can be recognized by others. We are at the present time engaged in exploring and understanding the common ground between us. We find that out of the confusion of human predicaments with which social workers are confronted there emerge certain essential truths about the people behind the predicaments and the ways in which help can be made available to them without loss of human dignity.

[1] *The Charity Organization Review*, No. 83, November, 1903.

It is on these essential matters, which have been extracted from knowledge and experience, and that are the concern of all social caseworkers, that the principles and techniques of casework practice are based. It is not my purpose here to discuss these principles in detail but I should like to say that from my point of view their validity is unquestioned because they reach down and give practical expression to the human rights which belong to us all, caseworkers and clients alike.

Having said this, I now want to take up my main theme, the question of agency function and its effect on the casework process. What does the agency do to the caseworker by putting him or her in a certain position in relation to the client, and how does this position affect the actual work done? These are, of course, complicated questions, and I want to try to formulate some preliminary ideas about them which may pave the way for further discussion. I shall make some general comments and then go on to discuss the work of three agencies, probation, child care, and medical social work.

I want to make it clear that I am not confusing agency function with agency policy or methods. I am concerned with the basic function of the agencies to meet social needs. We all know that policy and method can distort and obscure function and that only as all concerned can get a firm grip on function can this danger be avoided.

First of all I should like to say that I am aware that the casework principles which I have been referring to have been worked out and arrived at by workers in all kinds of agency settings and they are therefore not divorced from the influence of agency function on casework practice. They represent the common denominator of casework in all agencies whatever their function. As I have already implied, it seems to me important that we should not be so concerned with establishing our common casework skills based on commonly held principles that our view of the particular form in which problems are presented in our particular agency is obscured, otherwise we might fail to make full use of the function of our agency and of other agencies to meet the needs of clients. We must be confident enough in our common casework skills to be able to look at differences which exist between the agencies because of the particular function each has in relation to the client. In other words, although our function will be different according to the agency we are working in, our attitude to our clients and the ways in which we work with them will be the same whatever the agency.

Sometimes social workers talk as if the social services exist in order to provide a setting in which they can practice their casework skills. I can appreciate this keenness to establish professional skill—it must be present in every caseworker otherwise he or she will never achieve anything and moreover the drive to achieve means that the chosen profession gives scope for satisfactions in the individual. But the question of emphasis arises. Is the caseworker aiming at practising a professional skill, or at serving the community? We know that in the interests of all, these aims must be complementary and integrated into the professional life of each individual worker.

However, I do know that there are agencies which for all kinds of reasons do not give caseworkers the opportunity to develop their professional skills in the service of the agency. This may be a matter for adjustment between worker and agency. Such adjustment will take time, and it presents a challenge; or it may be, of course, that the agency needs structural alterations which will allow for the better deployment of staff resources as suggested for the health and welfare services in the Younghusband Report. But whatever the situation, I suggest that as we increasingly lay stress on the value of casework skill, it is important to remind ourselves that casework skill is not an end in itself, but is a means whereby we serve the community and find our place in it. I often wish that we were called social servants, because I think that this would describe our function today in a way that the term social worker does not. There is something dignified about being a servant, and moreover the word implies a relationship to the community whereas the word worker simply implies that work is being done.

At this point I should like to remind you of something that Professor Titmuss has said: 'the worker, the client, and the setting are the basic components of action and must be viewed as a whole.'[1] This statement seems to me to sum up much that is important for social workers. A sense of wholeness implies integration. If this sense of wholeness, which is necessary for maximum productivity, is missing we shall not be in a position to further the integration of our clients into the community, because at some point we ourselves have failed to achieve such an integration.

As social workers how do we become integrated into the community? Of course the ability to do this involves the achievement of maturity in the individual, a process which we know starts in the earliest years of life. It has been said that the hallmark of maturity is an individual's capacity to identify with the community without loss of identity and sense of self. I do not propose to trace the steps which

[1] 'The Administration Setting of Social Service', *Case Conference*, Vol. I, No. 1, May, 1954.

lead to this state of affairs now because they are very complex. But roughly speaking, if the needs of the individual are sufficiently well met at the various stages of development, then he or she comes to be able to identify with the people in the environment who meet his or her needs. Her own capacity to identify with her child is of course the basis of the mother's knowing what the child's needs are. This meeting of needs is a two-way process, a matter of giving and taking. The infant and child takes from his mother and at the same time gives to her her capacity to be a mother through her function as one, just as anyone who takes a present gives at the same time to the giver his capacity to give, to be a giver. This is what clients do for the social worker. By using our services they give us a function in relation to themselves and at the same time they give us a place in society which wants this function performed and has created the agency to perform it. Agency function therefore is not simply a meeting point for worker, client, and community, but a dynamic force which welds them together. It represents the creative urge in the community towards the client, and a creative urge in the client towards integration. These creative urges are embodied in the social worker who gives them 'vital meaning' in Professor Urwick's words. How vital the meaning will be will depend on the professional skill of the caseworker and on his or her own creativity. In my view therefore agency function is the central dynamic of the whole casework process. It is not something that is tacked on to casework and which is sometimes regarded as hampering to the practice of casework principles. It is the very crux of casework, and to lose touch with it would be to lose touch with the needs of our clients, and the forces in society which tend to meet these needs.

At this point I can imagine that some people may say this is all very well, but what about our difficult clients, those who seem beyond our scope and take and give nothing, and in whom the integrative urge is negligible? I think that this question does not really affect my argument, because the fact that they are our clients means that they are still within the scope of society's concern although we have as yet insufficient knowledge or provision to be able to help them. The less responsible the client can be, the more actively responsible must society become in relation to him through the function of its various social work agencies and their personnel. Obviously the majority of clients in any one agency are able to make use of the agency's function otherwise the agency would have died a natural death.

We all know that social work agencies can become obsolete. I like to remember that when I first started social work in what was then called a 'distressed area' I was concerned with something called 'The Mayor's Boot Fund' for unemployed miners. This agency obviously died long ago, for although presumably miners still need boots, they are no longer unemployed; and if they were, they come within the more effective national insurance policy which now exists.

As social conditions change the social needs of our clients express themselves in new forms which have to be recognized and understood in the light of new knowledge if the function of the agency in meeting needs is to be maintained. We recognize it as the special responsibility of the professionally trained social workers to keep under constant review, and to adjust to, the social needs of their clients, but the social workers are in a position to do this only because society employs them and in so doing takes the over-all responsibility for client and for worker alike.

How long society will go on taking this over-all responsibility depends on many factors, one of them undoubtedly being the social worker's ability not only to meet the needs of clients, but to contribute to the creating of a social climate in which the work will be maintained.

I should now like to apply what I have said about agency function in relation to casework by reference to the work of particular agencies.

First of all, probation. I was stimulated in my thinking about case-work in this setting by a paper given by Arthur Hunt, Principal Proba-tion Officer for Southampton in which he raised the problem of the application of casework techniques to probation work and particularly mentioned the important question of the compulsory nature of the relationship of the probation officer to his client. He says, 'The fact of enforcement has emerged as a much more positive feature than I would have believed at one time, and certainly more so than people are taught to expect, and is far from being an impediment to the application of casework techniques.'[1]

In view of what I have said about agency function it does not surprise me to find that Mr Hunt sees the enforced relationship as a positive factor in his work. In fact are there not theories which teach us that the delinquent is unconsciously looking for just this, for a human being to become a respected and controlling authority, because this is what he has been deprived of in his family relationships?

The clientele of the probation service mainly consists of boys and girls, men and women, who show a periodic exacerbation of an anti-social tendency which has become part of their lives. This tendency

[1] *Ventures in Professional Co-operation*, the Association of Psychiatric Social Workers, London, 1961.

belongs to a deprivation and repeats an urge (mainly unconscious), to reinstate what is lost. The individual steals in a claim over objects and satisfactions, or acts destructively expressing the unconscious need for a reinstatement of parental controls that have been absent at some crucial point or over a period of time.

When a child or an adult commits an offence of a certain degree and kind, he brings into action the machinery of the law. The probation officer who is then asked to do casework with the client feels he ought to apply techniques implying the casework principle of self-determination, but he loses everything if he forgets his relationship to his agency and the court, since symptoms of this kind of illness are unconsciously designed to bring authority into the picture. The probation officer can humanize the machinery of the law but he cannot side-step it without missing the whole point of the symptom and the needs of the client. If he does miss the point the client either gives up hope or commits another offence to ensure the reinstatement of legal machinery.[1]

In *The Probation Service* edited by Joan King[2] there is a story of a nine-year-old boy who after a few months surprised his officer by saying: 'It isn't reporting that matters'; and when asked what did matter, he replied: 'Yer promise to the Court.' Was not this child reaching out through the individual probation officer to feel the reality of the authority which the officer represented?

The principle of the client's right to self-determination is still implicit in the probation officer's work with his client, but the client will only be capable of becoming a self-determining individual if he finds a strongly backed environment in which he can safely live and discover his own true personal impulses.

There is then something deep down in the delinquent that comes to meet the probation officer, and this is why enforced relationships can work. It seems too that this is why the probation officer can often offer more to the delinquent than, for instance, the psychiatric or child guidance clinic. The delinquent may in fact need psychiatric treatment as well, but it cannot replace his primary need for a human being who is the embodiment of the legal machinery of society's reaction to him— a human being who is in a strong position in relation to himself and with whom he can gradually come to terms.

[1] See D. W. Winnicott, 'The Anti-Social Tendency', Collected Papers, Tavistock Publications, London, 1958.
John Bowlby, 'Forty-Four Juvenile Thieves', Balliere Tindall & Cox, London, 1946.
I am aware that sociological and other factors have a bearing on delinquency, but in my view these factors are of a secondary rather than a primary nature.
[2] Butterworth, London, 1958.

I suggest therefore that the probation officer finds that his agency's function reflects both the client's needs and society's reaction to these needs, and it also sets the basic pattern for the relationship. The effectiveness of the relationship will of course depend on the probation officer's ability to give vital meaning to the function, and in so doing his professional casework skills are fully needed.

I should now like to say something about the child care service, which is another legally backed social work agency with statutory obligations.

Roughly speaking its functions is a parental one, expressing the sense of responsibility that exists in the community towards children whose own parents are either temporarily or permanently unable to fulfil their obligations as parents. Behind the service is society's urge to meet the dependence needs of children. The service can therefore be regarded as preventive in respect of delinquency. Many kinds of social problems lie behind this fact of parental failure and the work will therefore vary accordingly. There will be the straightforward cases where illness, accident, death or other calamities have prevented the parents from functioning, but a considerable proportion will reveal the parents' personal immaturity arising from their own lack of satisfactory parental experiences. Sometimes the children must be provided with new parental figures and helped to accept them, sometimes by fulfilling a parental role in relation to the parents child care officers can enable them to maintain the care of their own children.

Agency function in the child care service therefore sets the basic pattern for the relationship between worker and client. The worker who performs the function embodies society's sense of parental responsibility towards the child who looks to her for just this. If a worker fails to embody the parental function of the agency in relation to the child, the child's needs will not be met. The worker does not of course become the child's parent in the day-to-day relationship which is concerned with his care and management, but she is the over-all caring parent behind the parents and the foster-parents, supporting their relationship and preserving continuity and reliability. As in probation, here again to side-step agency function would be to miss the point of the client's needs.

I know that trained caseworkers in the child care services sometimes find difficulty in reconciling their casework principles with the authoritative action that must sometimes be taken; for instance, action involving legal proceedings against parents who are seriously neglecting a child. A child care officer may have been working with these parents for a long time and although she may have helped them personally the child still suffers serious deprivation. Legal action seems to cut across the principle of the parents' right to self determination and of our acceptance of them as people, but in the interests of the child it must be taken. The child care officer feels a sense of failure, but she must be careful not to save herself from it by failing to take protective action on behalf of the child whose interests she alone in the situation represents. Moreover authoritative action, although it seems to cut across the casework relationship, can often be a relief because it makes the relationship more real, and strengthens it and often leads to more productive work.

Sometimes with adolescents in care it is difficult for the child care officer to know when the rights of the boy or girl to exercise self-determination must be over-ridden by the taking of direct responsibility for them. This is a tricky business, and indeed it is for parents in their own homes with their own children.

The child care officer with her wider experience and over-all knowledge of the total situation can often see that the self-determining behaviour of the adolescent is really cutting across his or her own best interests. The exercising of parental care which includes the taking of responsibility then surely becomes an obligation. A sixteen-year-old girl who was being difficult in a good foster-home where she was being tolerated. The difficulties arose because the girl was determined to leave this home and live with another couple who were trying to seduce her into this course of action. To cut a long story short, this other home was found to be unsuitable and the girl was told by the child care officer that after careful consideration it had been decided that she must stay in her present foster-home. There followed the expected outburst of tears, abuse, and difficult behaviour. But a week later something unexpected happened; when the child care officer visited she found the girl welcoming and friendly, and in a long interview talked more than she had ever done before of her feelings about her own mother, actually saying that when her mother told her to do something, for instance, go to bed at a certain time, she never went on to insist that the girl obeyed 'because she doesn't really care what happens to me'. The implication is obvious. The girl felt that the child care officer did care for her, and gradually with help she settled into the foster-home. By exercising the agency's function in relation to this child, a real need was met, and the casework relationship became much more meaningful.

I should now like to discuss medical social work. As I see it, the almoner's function is to enable the patient to make the fullest use of the medical care and treatment necessitated by his illness and to facilitate his recovery and readjustment to ordinary life.

I should like to quote a paragraph from the statement on medical social work prepared by the Institute of Almoners:

'Doctors have found that illness is often precipitated, intensified and prolonged by stresses and crises in a patient's personal life and environment, and unless prevented or relieved these difficulties may obstruct or even negate the value of treatment. Social casework contributes to medical care in hospital or home through a skilled appraisal of the source and significance of the social, emotional and economic complications of a patient's illness. It is needed in a medical setting because illness and disablement so often complicate people's lives. The recognition of medical social problems and the selection of patients who need social help is a matter requiring close co-operation between doctor and almoner. The doctor asks for the almoner's help when he considers that the patient has some personal family or environmental problems which have a bearing on the diagnosis or may influence the course of treatment.'

The almoner's function then is an integral part of the total function of the medical services, concerned with the patient's treatment and recovery, and the strength of her position in relation to a patient seems to me to lie in this fact. The patient endows the medical team with all kinds of powers for good or ill. His feelings about them are complicated by his hopes and his fears, by his expectations and his suspicions. As the member of the team specially trained to understand these feelings, the almoner can enable the patient to express them if he needs to do so. If she as a member of the team shows that she can identify with the patient by understanding his feelings and penetrating the sense of isolation which illness can impose, then he can through her identify with all who are trying to help him in the present situation, and can more readily co-operate in his own treatment and recovery. The almoner's agency function has put her in the position to help her client, but the quality of her casework skill will determine the effectiveness of her work.

I am not forgetting that not all patients will need casework help in this way, but many will have social problems connected with their illness and recovery and need practical help and advice. Here again the almoner because of her knowledge of the medical and social needs of the patient is in a position to enable him to use the services and provisions which exist both in her own setting and in other social agencies to help him. So the almoner's agency gives her a place to start from in the work of enabling the patient to co-operate in his own treatment.

It seems to me that what I have been saying about agency function implies something which needs to be explicit in our thinking. In functioning within an agency, a social caseworker as well as being a trained professional person who uses her knowledge and skill to help people, also becomes something in relation to her clients on behalf of the whole community. The probation officer becomes an authority figure, the child care officer becomes a parental figure, and the medical social worker as part of the medical team becomes a healing person on whom the patient's health depends.

If we fail to embody these roles in our work with our clients, something very vital will be lost. We shall in fact fail our clients at the point of their deepest need, which is to reintegrate through the services of the agency into the life of the community as independent self-determining people.

It would be profitable in my view to go on to consider the function of each of the other social work agencies and its effect on the casework process. In particular it would be interesting to compare the differences in this respect between the statutory and the voluntary agencies. Some important differences might be revealed which would throw light on the social work field as a whole. But that is a matter for another time and for further study.

To conclude I should like to repeat Professor Urwick's words of 1903 because they so succinctly express what I have been trying to say. '... [The Social Worker] must learn to see in the social structure whole or part, of state or of institution, the expression of a vital meaning.'

8

CO-ORDINATION REVIEWED*

OLIVE STEVENSON

SOME of us have been feeling recently that the topic of co-ordination and co-operation in social work has become a little stale. Everyone agrees it is a good and necessary thing but the suggestions made to explain why it is only partially successful seem to have been for the most part superficial. The Ingleby Committee[1] referred to 'interdepartmental rivalries' and having bitten on such a gristly topic, choked and said no more. I would like to look more deeply at a few of the difficulties involved, acknowledging from the outset that many aspects of the subject will be untouched or insufficiently explored. For example, I do not propose to take up the Ingleby contention that many of the problems are due to failure to distinguish between the processes involved—the processes of 'detection, investigation and treatment'. My own view is that this is not a particularly helpful line of enquiry.

The Oxford Dictionary defines co-ordination as: 'the harmonious combination of agents or functions towards the production of a result.' The last phrase of this definition is interesting—'towards the production of a result.' One can profitably ask the question—is there one desired result in a problem of co-ordination? But this I will return to later.

To clarify and focus our thinking, here is an example of a familiar type of co-ordinating committee:

It is a July day in Southdown in the Town Hall; in a small committee room decorated in beige and chocolate brown the co-ordinating committee sits. The following are present:

The children's officer (Chairman).
The child care officer.
The medical officer of health.

* *Case Conference*, Vol. IX, No. 8, February, 1963.
[1] *Report of the Committee on Children & Young Persons*, H.M.S.O., London, 1960.

H

The health visitor.
The mental welfare officer.
The probation officer.
The national assistance board officer.
The housing manager.

The Long family is being discussed: they are living in very poor conditions in privately owned property; they have four children, two under five. The mother is mentally ill, usually rather depressed, she has periods in hospital in acute phases. Psychiatric reports suggest that the position is unlikely to change in the foreseeable future. The father is frequently unemployed: he is on probation for theft of coal from a nearby merchant's yard. There is no previous history of delinquency. The children are poorly fed and clothed and the general conditions are dirty. It is obvious to everyone that despite all this the family ties are strong. The meeting has been called by the medical officer of health because of his concern and that of the health visitor, over the home conditions and the housing manager has been invited to see if there is any possibility of re-housing the Longs in council property.

I have deliberately chosen a fairly commonplace example with no outstandingly unusual features. Now let us consider what often happens at such a meeting. Our definition of co-ordination concludes that it is 'towards the production of a result'. What is the desired result of the members of this committee for the Long family? Can it be described by a fine sounding phrase like—'the well-being of the family in society'? A general statement of this kind glosses over all kinds of conflicts which I shall try to analyse below. In fact this co-ordinating committee consists of people with a diversity of aims and emphases, all of which at their best are laudable, none of which is totally opposed. Nevertheless there are real problems of balance.

The housing manager and the National Assistance Board officer may see themselves to a greater extent than the others present as guardians of society's resources; not concerned primarily with this family but preoccupied with their responsibility to society as a whole—that the taxpayers shall not be exploited, that the needs of others beside the Longs for houses shall be emphasized. Beneath this may be a deep and urgent desire that some system of external fairness shall be preserved and 'justice shall be seen to be done'. Of course no social worker can afford to ignore this issue but we are speaking of differing emphases, not absolute distinctions, and the focus of the social workers present will inevitably be on the Longs—on their need for decent housing to help improve their standards. The point is perhaps more subtly illustrated by the conflict which arises between the probation officer and the National Assistance Board officer concerning Mr Long's poor work record. This is seen by the National Assistance Board officer as a wilful refusal to get and keep employment and it is felt to be quite wrong that such a man should be supported by the state. The probation officer, while wishing that Mr Long would go to work, sees it as indicative of the total family problem; he believes that Mrs Long's depression makes it extremely difficult for her husband to leave her alone with the children and that on balance it may be best that Mr Long should remain at home most of the time.

It is sometimes extremely difficult to disentangle the various issues involved in such a discussion—which we can hear any day of the week between the social worker and those who do not see themselves primarily as social workers but who are nevertheless much involved with the social services. Obviously it is in part a matter of knowledge and understanding of human beings. But is this all? Can and should the National Assistance Board officer, knowing more of the dynamics of the Long family, decide that Mr Long need not work? Should the housing manager, understanding the effect that dreary housing conditions are having on this mother's depressed and apathetic state, rehouse the Longs over the heads of 100 other families less urgently in need but longer on the list and causing no problem to the social workers? We may have to take care that we do not punish the deserving.

One can of course discern the psychological factors which affect such discussions. The identifications and the personal problems of the participants are often clear. Beneath the arguments that Mr Long 'ought' to work may lurk punishing attitudes, not uncommonly found in those whose own sense of duty is harsh, and based on fear rather than love. The probation officer's arguments may reflect a sympathy with the underdog, even a collusion with him against authority. Nevertheless to point this out is not to dispose of a real social problem of judgement and decision in weighing up the needs of the Long family with the needs of other families and the rights of society to defend itself against exploitation. There is no one answer to this problem; it is rather a matter of preserving a healthy tension, with as much personal insight as possible.

This then is our first point of conflict in this co-ordinating committee. It would be simple indeed if the problems ended there but this is only one of a series of cross currents. At a field work level, one can discern two types of difficulty—not completely separate, of course, but different enough to be considered apart. These are, firstly, differences in method; secondly, differences of function and involvement.

Amongst those who can be considered as social caseworkers at this committee there will be marked differences of method and skill in the understanding and treatment of people. Furthermore, those who do not consider themselves social caseworkers may be puzzled and even threatened by the approach of the caseworker. There are problems here both of general education and also of professional training with which everyone is familiar and upon which I do not wish to dwell. In practice, one of the most common causes of friction turns on casework method; granted everyone wants the Longs to clean up their house and care for their children better—how best to achieve it? In this case, the child care officer has been visiting regularly; she happens (though this would by no means always be the case) to be a qualified professional caseworker. With the bloom of a generic course still fresh upon her, she has firmly in mind two basic casework assumptions: 'start where the client is' and 'the value of advice-giving is limited'. She upholds these in her work with Mrs Long. She accepts Mrs Long's depression as a fact and believes that she must start there; she does not exhort her to cheer up or to clean up since she believes it would only make Mrs Long feel less and less adequate as a wife and mother, already she is drowned in self reproaches and guilt characteristic of the depressive. All this is, however, upsetting to the health visitor. Her training as a nurse has made her sensitive to the harm done to the children by poor nutrition, dirty conditions and so on. She wants action, and so does her medical officer of health, to improve this situation speedily. The child care officer does not think this can be effective. There are conflicts of method in the actual help this mother receives from the child care officer and health visitor who both visit. This shows at the meeting when the medical officer of health acidly remarks that 'deep casework' seems to mean visiting for years and talking about anything rather than the actual problem of a dirty house and dirty children.

I have chosen to compare the child care officer and the health visitor; but it could of course have been different services, depending on the area; it is inevitable that in this stage of rapid development in social work in this country we should find these difficulties in understanding the objectives and methods of others. The value of more recent developments in casework method is not yet proven; also, behind criticism there may be envy. Sometimes there is imperfect understanding by the untrained social worker of what may reasonably be hoped for from the trained caseworker. Idealization and denigration are two sides of the same coin, both equally unreal. We see today something of the same attitudes to caseworkers as are found towards psychiatrists. Casework is either black or white magic, it can solve nothing or solve everything.

I have linked the words function and involvement since in day-to-day practice they are inseparable, as Clare Winnicott's recent article on agency function has shown. [1] In discussion, however, one can separate them; by functions I mean those duties laid upon a social worker by the agency and by involvement I mean the inner feelings of the worker towards particular clients and their needs.

Returning to the Long's, let us look at these problems. The mental welfare officer has helped Mrs Long in her various phases of acute depression prior to her admission to hospital. Since the Mental Health Act, 1959, the psychiatrists in the hospital have laid increasing emphasis on the care of the mentally ill in the community. The mental welfare officer believes that his patient is best at home for as often and as long as possible. He sees that there are real dangers of a kind of apathetic institutionalization; but he also recognizes that there are strains in all this for the family. The probation officer believes strongly that it is an intolerable burden for Mr Long to have his wife at home in this condition and would prefer that Mrs Long should have longer spells in hospital. He feels it might be best for the children to be received into care. The child care officer is also deeply concerned about the effect of mental illness on these children, especially as the older ones have to shoulder responsibility beyond their years. But she knows, as no one else at the meeting, that being in care is no picnic; that warm foster mothers do not always materialize; that the ties of children to their home may be overwhelmingly strong, whether healthy or neurotic. Part of these difficulties arise from actual knowledge in the possession of the one that the others do not have. But there is much that goes deeper. As we all know, the structure of our social services has tended to give particular social workers a bit of the family to be concerned about especially. Obviously this can be modified by knowledge of other responsibilities, by increasing emphasis on the family as a whole—both of which are affected by education and training. Even so, there remains the personal and inward identification of the worker; sometimes, though not necessarily, reinforced by the agency's function. This point comes out clearly at the co-ordinating committee. The mental welfare officer, a large, kindly man, feels most protective towards Mrs Long, so timid and pathetic, and this fits in happily with the focus of his work. The health

[1] Clare Winnicott, 'Casework and Agency Function', *Case Conference*, Vol. VIII, No. 7, January, 1962.

visitor, an energetic woman who has overcome many obstacles in her own life, is intolerant of Mrs Long's hopelessness and both inwardly, and by reason of her professional concern with the under fives, is child-focused. It is, of course, quite possible that the personal identification might differ from the agency identification and this must often occur. In this connection however one has to recognize the unconscious drives that cause us at times to select one branch of social work rather than another.

All this assumes that conflicts may arise between the needs of different people within the family. One may argue that ultimately the needs of individuals within the family are going to be the same and usually in the long term this will be so; the rescuing of children from the unsatisfactory parents is an example of short term action which has often proved in the long term to be disastrous. Nevertheless, we must not glibly pass over the fact that the family unit, locked together as it is, nevertheless contains separate people with separate needs and rights. This is particularly important where mental illness is concerned. This may have to be seen in terms of both partners need for the illness, but in Mrs Long's case, her feeling for her children seems at times to reflect her need to be kept alive by them rather than her capacity to give in love. In her depression she feels dead inside and the children are a live bit of her to which she clings. In them their mother's sadness provokes considerable guilt and anxiety. One must seek first to identify and weigh up such factors before one can begin to make appropriate plans. If there has to be a choice between the needs, for instance, of the mother and the children, one can be helped to a decision by the fact the children may be helped to break out of a vicious circle which will otherwise be perpetuated to the next generation, but this is always a painful decision and one in which frictions between social workers are likely to occur.

The involvement of the social worker with a particular member of the family does pose considerable problems for a co-ordinating committee. Yet there are still other kinds of involvement. The very problems for example, of debt and dirt, or of parental roles, which the Long family, and many others, present, are those which rouse deep feeling in the workers, intimately concerned as they are with social and psychological attitudes, built up within us over the years. It is inevitable that for different workers different problems will seem more pressing or more disturbing than others, and this will add to the tensions in co-ordination. The controversy between the National Assistance Board officer and the probation officer about Mr Long's unemployment is sharpened by the feeling of the National Assistance Board officer that

Mr Long's almost feminine role in the home is inappropriate and even unhealthy.

So far the problems of co-ordination have been considered at the field work level; the role of the higher grades of administration in the process remain to be discussed.

One often hears that co-operation is satisfactory at the field work level, it's the chief officers that make it difficult. 'If they would leave us alone, we would get on all right.' A simple and obvious fact must first be faced. Senior officers should have obtained their posts by reason of special ability which shouuld include a capacity to analyse, clarify and synthesize issues, which is clearly of vital importance in the guidance of a co-ordinating committee. There is unfortunately no doubt that this capacity is frequently lacking. The motive which we loosely describe as empire-building also enters into the difficulties and the desire for power is a common feature in the higher levels of organization. It is sad that the basic question 'Who can serve this client best?' is often lost sight of in the midst of rivalries which at the present time are often focused on the question—'Who should do preventive work?' Problems such as the health visitor and child care officer experienced in the Long case over casework method may be taken up and used by chief officers. On these issues, opinions may be rationally held and cogent arguments advanced on either side. But they are frequently complicated by other less wholesome motives. Simon's book: *Administrative Behavior* studies many different factors involved in decision making in any organization. He makes the point that identification with an organization is necessary in order to cope with the problem of rational choice. 'Identification is an important mechanism for constructing the environment of decision.'[1] This is because it limits the issues which the people concerned have to consider and cope with. Simon suggests, however, that the high-level administrator must have wider horizons:

'Observation indicates that, as the higher levels are approached in adminstrative organizations, the administrator's 'internal' task (his relations with the organization subordinate to him) decreases in importance relative to his 'external' task (his relations with persons outside the organization). An ever larger part of his work may be subsumed under the heads of 'public relations' and 'promotion'. The habits of mind characteristic of the administrative roles at the lower and higher levels of an organization undoubtedly show differences corresponding to these differences in function.

[1] Herbert A. Simon, *Administrative Behavior* (2nd edit.), Macmillan Company, New York, 1960, p. 211.

'At the lower levels of the hierarchy, the frame of reference within which decision is to take place is largely given. The factors to be evaluated have already been enumerated, and all that remains is to determine their values under the given circumstances. At the higher levels of the hierarchy, the task is an artistic and an inventive one. New values must be sought out and weighed; the possibilities of new administrative structures evaluated. The very framework of reference within which decision is to take place must be constructed.

'It is at these higher levels that organizational identifications may have their most serious consequences. At the lower level, the identification is instrumental in bringing broad considerations to bear on individual situations. It ensures that decisions will be made responsibly and impersonally. At the higher levels, identifications serve to predetermine the decision, and to introduce among its assumptions unrecognized and unverified valuations.'[1]

Thus, in our sphere of interest Simon would place fairly and squarely on the chief officers' shoulders' the task of looking beyond the confines of his own organization towards the wider values and objectives of the social services as a whole. Sectional loyalties, one may feel, are inevitable and even necessary at the field work level but at the higher levels one should have different expectations. One must recognize that at the present time, for a variety of reasons, not all senior officers are of the calibre, intellectually and professionally, to fulfil these functions in relation to co-ordination. It happens not infrequently that field workers are better qualified than their senior officers which means that the former lack the informed support which is their right in any organization. Simon's comments point up the great need in social work at the present time to study at greater depth the administrative processes.

To summarise: one may I think group the difficulties of co-ordination under four general heads: firstly, problems of social philosophy; secondly, of casework skills; thirdly, of the workers' function and involvement; fourthly, of the administrator's role. Only by a circular and complicated route like this, can we find our way back again to the Long family, to the family in need, whom we so often fail through our clouded perception of the processes in which we are involved. In all that is discovered, two essentials will I believe emerge, the need for deeper personal insight, on the one hand, and on the other, the need for wider vision of the objectives of the social services as a whole.

[1] Op cit., pp. 217–18.

9

TREATMENT OF CHARACTER DISORDERS: A DILEMMA IN CASEWORK CULTURE*

OTTO POLLAK

In the treatment of character disorders, social caseworkers deal with three groups of difficulties. The first concerns the nature of the condition itself. The main difficulty in work with persons with character disorders is that, because of the primitive ego structure of the persons afflicted, the therapist and the client must engage not only in a process of unlearning faulty reaction patterns but also in a process of diversification and creation in social development. Clients require a type of therapy which emphasizes psychological nurture more than gains in understanding, identification with the ego of the therapist, and therefore acceptance of limitations rather than liberation from maladaptive restrictions. Sometimes the course of therapy shows movement even through the development of a neurosis as a step towards health.[1]

Second, the nature of our civilization not only seems to elicit the development of character disorders in an increasing number of people but it also lends support to the persistence of such disorders. From individualism to egotism there is only one step. From romantic love to unrealistic expectations regarding gratifications that can be demanded from the marriage partner there is equally only one. And from such unrealistic expectations to the limitation of one's own giving and the resultant violation of reciprocity in marital interaction the distance is not long either. In a materialistic society, id-gratifications are prominently offered in overt and hidden form, while the waning power of a generally accepted morality leaves superego forces unsupported. That under such

* Published in *The Social Service Review*, Vol. XXXV, No. 2, June, 1961.
[1] Rosemary Reynolds and Else Siegle, 'A Study of Casework with Sadomasochistic Marriage Partners', *Social Casework*, Vol. XL, December, 1959, pp. 545–51; Effie Warren, 'Treatment of Marriage Partners with Character Disorders', *Social Casework*, Vol. XXXVIII, March, 1957, pp. 118–26; and Otto Pollak, Hazel M. Young, and Helen Leach, 'Differential Diagnosis and Treatment of Character Disturbances', *Social Casework*, Vol. XLI, December, 1960, pp. 512–17.

conditions all compromise between id and superego should be weighted on the id side need not be surprising. Most of all, however, a society that mistrusts authority and extols rebellion is likely to furnish many rationalizations to a person whose psychic structure leads to acting-out rather than to internalization of conflict.[1] In this cultural framework, psycho-analysis, with its liberating impact upon conventional restrictions in the expressions of sexuality and hostility, has become over-extended in the popular mind. Our current civilization, therefore, continually feeds new strength into the resistiveness to treatment of clients who are afflicted with character disorders.

The third complex of difficulties which caseworkers encounter in their therapeutic efforts with this group of clients stems from their own professional culture. These difficulties will be presented here in hypothetical form as a basis for scrutiny and discussion by practitioners. The central thesis presented is that caseworkers have made their greatest professional advances in an orientation of theory and practice concerned with the treatment of the classic symptom neuroses and with character disturbances accompanied by guilt, while they are now faced with clients who exhibit character disturbances which are relatively guilt-free and which lead to conflict in interaction with other people rather than to intrapersonal conflict in the client. Caseworkers find themselves, therefore, sometimes entrapped by the principles of a method of casework which does not appear appropriate for the new group of clients who seem to dominate the case loads of family welfare agencies today. Apparently every success in fighting discomforts in the social sphere is followed by new discomforts which could not have been foreseen. Success in the fight against infant mortality necessitated increased concern with the management of sensory disorders which survived perinatal injuries. The gain in survival of the middle-aged has brought into focus the problems of degenerative diseases. And apparently our successful fight against the symptom neuroses has increased our difficulties in finding means of effective treatment of character disorders.

In order to clarify the nature of these difficulties, it may be helpful to describe the syndrome from which clients with character disorders seem to suffer. The constellation commonly described as a character disorder, as distinguished from a character neurosis, seems to present a constellation of massive projection, ego-syntonic behaviour, insistence on self-justification and the need for change in others, insensitivity to the needs

[1] Otto Pollak, 'Social Factors Contributing to Character Disorders', *Child Welfare*, Vol. XXXVII, April, 1958, pp. 8–12.

of others, hopelessness, and inefficient exploitation of others.[1] Mere inspection of this constellation of characteristics will suggest that casework help oriented to guilt and discomfort in self-perception will find itself without points of easy contact with clients so afflicted. It may serve, however, the task of reorientation which diagnostically oriented casework requires if the difficulties in this respect are elaborated and analysed. That 'therapeutic techniques that are effective with neurotic clients are not appropriate with character disorders'[2] has been clearly recognized and frequently stated in the literature. What has to be elaborated and presented to the profession is the fact that the principles of casework appropriate for the treatment of neurotic clients have by and large been generalized in the subculture of the profession so that principles appropriate for the treatment of character disorders present problems in the professional culture as it has developed. These difficulties will be presented under the headings of relationship difficulties, difficulties in setting goals, and difficulties in treatment methods.

The outstanding difficulty in establishing a positive relationship with clients afflicted with character disorders stems from the fact that the professional training and experience of social caseworkers produce a personality which is the opposite of the personality encountered in such clients. A high degree of self-awareness, sensitivity to the nature of his interactions with others, and ability to give of himself for the benefit of others are the attributes which we find and welcome in successful caseworkers. The client suffering from the impact of a character disorder upon his relationships with others is a person who uses projection, is insensitive to the need of others, and is unable to give in interaction with others. Since the essential quality of a positive relationship is a feeling of 'at-oneness'[3] with somebody else, it can easily be recognized that there will be difficulties in the initial interaction between the caseworker and such clients. Opposites have little chance to establish rapport from the start. It is therefore understandable that Effie Warren has found it necessary to publish a warning to caseworkers against the temptation to expect such clients to volunteer facts about their own part in the marital relationships and to cut short such persons in the first interview by bringing them back to a consideration of their own

[1] Pollak, Young and Leach, op. cit., p. 513.

[2] Beatrice R. Simcox and Irving Kaufman, M.D., 'Treatment of Character Disorders in Parents of Delinquents', *Social Casework*, Vol. XXXVII, October, 1956, p. 388.

[3] Helen Harris Perlman, *Social Casework: A Problem-solving Process*, Chicago: University of Chicago Press, 1957, p. 66.

behaviour.[1] This, however, is only a consideration of the problem as far as the caseworker is concerned.

It is probable that the client also becomes consciously or unconsciously aware of the contradiction between his own personality and that of the caseworker. On the conscious level, at least, the very personality of the caseworker may present a reproach to the client with a character disorder. Very few of us are able to perceive a person as being helpful if he is very different or if he is actually the opposite of what we are. The client would much rather sense in a therapist a fellow sufferer than a person who is a stranger to his condition. On the other hand, the therapist probably finds it easier to treat a person whose condition he has experienced than one whose experience he has never known. Since self-selection, screening in admission interviews, and professional success in social casework probably have resulted in selection of personnel more inclined to neurosis that to character disorder, the sympathy created by similarity between therapist and client is unlikely to exist between the caseworker and the client with a character disorder. The only at-oneness which may come quickly is the id stimulation which the caseworker receives from the client, i.e. the acting-out stimulation, the vicarious gratification of receiving without giving, of expressing hostility and hoping to get away with it. Against this type of at-oneness the professional caseworker will be on guard, of course, but even being on guard presents a special strain and for that reason may be the cause of still another difficulty in establishing a positive relationship with this type of client.

Always exploiters of human relationships, clients with character disorders will be tempted to exploit the caseworker by using his skills for their pathological needs. Such clients have probably come to the agency because they have found their exploitative efforts in human relations ineffective. What they want is first of all an increase in the accessibility to exploitation in their marriage partners, or children. Unconsciously, at least, they want to become better exploiters rather than more giving persons. Even though they accept the need for self-change, they want most of all to free themselves only of those aspects of their behaviour which interfere with their raid on the personal resources of others. The caseworker will not be able to accept either of these goals and thus by professional conviction about health in human relationships will become in fact an opponent of the client. Casework culture extols reciprocity in human relationships; character disorder defies it.

The basic difference expresses itself also in an incongruity between

[1] Warren, op. cit., p. 120.

the perceptions of the client and the perceptions of the caseworker. As a result of the fruitful contact which social casework has had with dynamically oriented psychiatry, the professional perception of caseworkers is geared to individual diagnosis. The caseworkers wants to understand the client who presents himself to him as a person in a situation; the client with a character disorder perceives only his situation as unsatisfactory and is entirely concerned with the part that others play in his interpersonal relationships. The client sees what he does not get; the caseworker sees—largely—what the client does not give.

Within recent years the perception of caseworkers has shown signs of reorientation towards the diagnosis of interpersonal relationships and family groups. Yet all these understandings and diagnostic formulations are based on individual diagnoses of the persons involved. In consequence, it is extremely difficult for a caseworker to establish a common frame of reference with such clients from the start. Even, for instance, if the caseworker manages to keep in diagnostic focus two marriage partners with character disorders, the two will be concerned only with what they do not get while the caseworker will be concerned with what both of them do not give. This contest makes it difficult for the caseworker to establish a common goal with the client early in the contact, even though establishing such a common goal is elementary.[1]

The caseworker must learn to be patient with this client group and to be satisfied with agreement with the client on the desirability of certain sub goals which from the point of view of casework cannot be accepted as the sum total of desirability. In the last analysis, of course, the caseworker must see the goal in such cases in the capacity of the client to meet the needs of others. The suggestion made by Rosemary Reynolds and Else Siegle[2]—to connect with the client's narcissism in a logical discussion of behaviour changes which will make things easier for him—presents for the caseworker the difficulty of trying to use a condition in the client which represents immaturity and pathology. In this respect some reorientation will probably be necessary to make the suggestion by Reynolds and Siegle an easily workable procedure. The solution may lie in the proposition that maturity and immaturity are designations of conditions which in their purity are unlikely to be found in clients. People are more or less geared to reciprocity, more or less self-concerned, and the caseworker must learn to use the client's potential in these respects without the mental reservation that he is

[1] Lenore Rivesman, 'Casework Treatment of Severely Disturbed Marriage Partners', Social Casework, Vol. XXXVIII, May, 1957, p. 244.
[2] Reynolds and Siegle, op. cit., p. 549.

actually fostering the undesirable or is arresting the client's development.

Perhaps most significant, however, is the fact that clients with character disorders are prone to attacks of depression and hopelessness which make them need persistent encouragement and support from the caseworker. In this respect the culture of casework makes the helping task difficult. Caseworkers notoriously underestimate their effectiveness and are therefore cautious in predicting or promising significant improvement to the clients. It might be worth investigating how many cases are lost after one or two contacts simply because caseworkers hesitate to hold out definite hope to depressive clients. While it may be impossible, because of the nature of the condition, to establish with the client a framework of common understanding and common goals, it may be possible to establish with him a framework of common expectations regarding his improvement and to renew such a framework when the client has a relapse into depressive moods.

There is no aspect of the helping process in which the culture conflict between a caseworker and the client with character disorder expresses itself more clearly than in treatment goals. If it is correct, as is often assumed, that most therapists have a neurotic personality basis, then it is within their own professional and, perhaps, therapeutic experience that the treatment process is liberating rather than binding. Guilt and anxiety are decreased, spontaneity is increased, self-blame and self-restriction are eased. The client with a character disorder, however, brings to the casework process a personality structure which requires binding instead of liberation, the creation of a measure of guilt and anxiety rather than emotional release from such conditions, restriction of behaviour in place of maladaptive spontaneity. To the caseworker who considers these treatment goals it must look therefore as if he were about to take from the client something which he, the worker, has achieved at the price of great effort and emotional investment. People who have become liberated find themselves in a position in which they are to set up limitations for the client and in which they have to help the client towards an internalization of limitations.

In the treatment of character disorders, there is a surface implication of taking away rather than of giving which is in direct contradiction not only with the culture of casework but with our culture in general. Having grown out of material giving, casework still wants to 'give' to the client in emotional and psychological respects. Actually, treatment methods appropriate in character disorders demand more such giving than any other type of diagnostically oriented casework, but this giving is method, not goal. The goal is one of taking away from the client his spontaneity in acting out his needs for gratification and expression, his freedom from guilt, his unconcern with others. What the worker does take away from the client in goal-setting is something which we all somewhat regret that we have lost in our upbringing and development, freedom for the id.

Furthermore, social caseworkers sometimes are still under the impact of the goal definition in the *Report on Scope and Methods* of the Family Service Association of America which was formulated with an orientation to people suffering from an excess of guilt and the resulting disabling conditions. It will be remembered that the report identified two treatment aims of social casework: (1) to support and maintain the client's current strengths by helping him to mobilize capacity and resources to meet his current life-situation, and (2) to modify the client's attitudes and patterns of behaviour by increasing his understanding of himself, of his problems, and of his part in creating them.[1] Neither of these two aims seems to meet the needs of the client with a character disorder. Support and maintenance of his strength are not appropriate because the client does not have enough strength. In modifying attitudes through increased understanding, the emphasis is on cognition; the client is to be helped to become the scholar of his misery. In the character disorder, on the other hand, treatment aims at more than either of these goals suggests. It aims at growth of motivation. To achieve this requires a much greater investment by the caseworker than helping the client to maintain strength or to increase understanding. The report is an invitation to do either too much too soon or not enough. What the client with a character disorder needs is, to borrow a term from computer language, 'input' which will enable him in the long run to produce emotional and interpersonal 'output'. He must be invested in to become able to pay interpersonal dividends. Before such an investment is fully made, understanding will not be accessible to him, and what glimpses of understanding he may gain will probably be abused as the rationalization of further acting-out. In terms of goals, then understanding will never be enough to help these clients; before they can become able to gain understanding they must be motivated to interact with others in a giving rather than in an exploiting way.

As far as treatment methods are concerned, the life-history approach, particularly the dwelling upon childhood experiences, is likely to prove of doubtful therapeutic value. Eliciting of childhood experiences and

[1] *The Scope and Methods of the Family Service Agency: Report of the Committee on Methods and Scope*, Family Service Association of America, New York, 1953, p. 7.

the feelings which accompanied them is necessary for liberation from morbid anxieties, but it is not indicated for the creation of a readiness in the client to accept limitations and restrictions. In the person with a character disorder there is nothing to be gotten rid of because there is not enough there. Delving into the past can bring the client into stronger contact with his id impulses. What is appropriate in order to undo the impact of an overstrict overego is contraindicated in the absence of an adequately developed one. In a way both client and caseworker are deprived of the intellectual gratification resulting from a genetic diagnosis. Since this gratification, however, would furnish for the client only justification for his non-giving and exploitative behaviour, the caseworker in turn must learn to get along without it.

If caseworkers are concerned about a relatively low degree of success in work with character disorders, they must remind themselves that they start with many handicaps created by past learning. Perhaps one of the outstanding therapeutic reaction patterns which caseworkers have had to learn is permissiveness. In a world in which everybody has evaluated the client and has shown him various degrees of dissatisfaction with his performance, the at least overtly non-critical attitude of the caseworker has made it easy for the client to distinguish between therapist on the one hand and spouse, parent, employer, and members of the peer group on the other. In the treatment of character disorders this clear-cut differentiation is likely to be lost. Since a strong element of nurture and personality rearing has to be incorporated into the therapeutic effort, the setting of norms and limits, at least indirectly and later on directly, has to enter the complex of therapeutic interaction with the client.

'Rearing' demands more giving—and more denying—than conventional therapy, be it supportive therapy, clarification, or insight therapy. Along with permissiveness, the caseworker must abandon inactivity. Clients with character disorders require praise for even very minor achievement, for sporadic even if abortive effort. When they break appointments, they require more reaching-out from the caseworker than a simple letter or a telephone call. They require sensitivity and response to their hopelessness; they require advice and guidance.[1]

On the other hand, there are certain conventional patterns of casework influence which seem inappropriate. Feelings are not to be elicited because the client already suffers from too great a flow of feeling into action. He is 'acting-out' and suffers the consequences. To release his feelings further and thus to increase his acting-out might bring him

---

[1] Warren, op. cit., p. 213; Reynolds and Siegle, op. cit., p. 549.

into conflict with the authorities, might lead to the breakup of his marriage, or might induce panic.

Setting limits, on the other hand, may furnish an easy cover for the counter transference of the caseworker. Since these are clients who are likely to tax the potential of the caseworker for empathy, counter transference is perhaps a greater danger here than in the treatment of other types of pathology. To be forced into a limit-setting relationship by the nature of the disorder is likely to make it more difficult for the caseworker to become aware of the emergence of non-therapeutic reactions on his part to the client.

There is also the trying demand for prolonged—and renewed—therapy which the elements of nurture and rearing in this type of treatment present. Our general culture has come to value speed as a sign of efficiency. Casework, as well as psychiatric treatment, has not remained unaffected by this tendency. Treatment of clients with character disorders, however, does last longer and moves less perceptibly than even long-term treatment which caseworkers, who do not yield easily to cultural pressure, have defined as standard.

The caseworker who has read this paper may well be left with the following impressions: (1) that he has heard all these treatment suggestions before, and (2) that there is no peace on the development of treatment techniques and of theoretical clarifications. Both impressions are correct, but the implications of fatigue and impatience which they carry may be based on an erroneous assumption. It has always been part of our culture to believe that one final effort might free us from burdensome aspects of human existence. We accept war only as a means to end all wars. We buy blue chips in order to be able to forget all about them. We court a person who might make a desirable mate and after marriage abandon efforts to further his affection and positive responses. In reality there is no peace and there are no final solutions. Every effort creates new problems, and every solution of these problems creates new ones in turn. Caseworkers appear frequently to be exhorted to return to methods of treatment and to approaches which one or two decades ago they were called upon to abandon. Such exhortations are not recantations, they are not the abandonment of fads, they are not the expressions of artificial obsolescence. The ability of the helping professions to remain aware of the swings of the social pendulum and to be able to respond to them seems to be the sign of a high degree of professional maturity.

I

10

EGO DEFICIENCY IN DELINQUENTS *

HYMAN GROSSBARD

DELINQUENCY is a complex phenomenon that takes many forms and stems from a myriad of interacting forces. In spite of the complexity of the phenomenon, however, I shall endeavour to identify some of the common elements in the personality structures and adaptive mechanisms of delinquents. I shall not attempt to analyse sociocultural factors in the genesis or treatment of delinquent behaviour, but shall limit my discussion to personality factors.

Most delinquents have patterns of behaviour that are indicative of basic disturbances in personality structure. In many instances the nature of these disturbances leads to a diagnosis of character disorder. The term character disorder suggests that an all-pervasive disturbance affects the individual's total behaviour. Although this term is an apt description, it does not illuminate sufficiently the dynamics of the psychological processes. In order to understand the idiosyncrasies of the delinquent with a character disorder, it is necessary to appraise the total psyche and its various components. The same procedure, of course, is necessary for a delinquent with other types of psychological disturbance. It is my belief that all delinquents, regardless of the type of disturbance, have certain common psychological processes that operate vertically in their history and horizontally in their functioning.

The search for common elements in delinquent behaviour must begin with an analysis of the formation and functioning of the ego, the psyche's most important agent for dealing with reality. My experience in the direct treatment of delinquents has led me to believe that understanding of the individual's ego mechanisms is central to effective treatment. The delinquent has inefficient ego mechanisms, and as a result he tends to act out conflict rather than to handle it by rational means or by symptom formation. A number of these inefficient ego mechanisms will be described.

* Published in *Social Casework*, Vol. XLIII, No. 4, April, 1962.

A basic ego function is to develop mechanisms of control to deal with both internal and external stimuli. These control mechanisms evolve as a result of a complex set of processes; these processes, in turn, facilitate the development of additional mechanisms and more-advanced modes of behaviour. The delinquent usually has little ability to tolerate frustration, to control his responses to stimuli, or to postpone gratification. Insufficient attention has been given to the nature and extent of these deficiencies. We tend to think of controls as conscious processes whereas in reality they evolve from, and begin to function on, the unconscious level. By transformation and conversion, infantile controls subsequently evolve into the more advanced controls of language and symbols. Thus the ego delays, freezes, and masters id drives as they go through the process of reaching the ideational and conscious level.

The delinquent, however, continues to act out his id drives, using activity rather than language to cope with his impulses. His ego is unable to channel his id impulses into the acceptable grooves of language and symbols. His drives spill over; they permeate his whole body and are expressed in hyperactivity and restlessness. He discharges tension through activity rather than verbalization. He is not unlike the infant who dissipates his tensions through direct actions, such as kicking and crying. In the process of growing up he does not develop the usual distance between his wishes and the expression of them.

Since the ego function of translating desires into language and thereby binding and delaying them is lacking in the delinquent, he is deprived of a significant form of control and mastery. A person with more advanced ego development is able to recognize the source of an irritation and convert the irritation into a conscious plan for relieving it. If he is hungry, he begins to wish for food and to think of ways of satisfying his hunger. Converting a wish into an idea gives the wish shape and form, robbing it of its frightening infinity. Identifying the source of irritation opens the way to finding a source of relief. It is through these processes that an individual learns how to master impulses.

The possible ways of harnessing, delaying, and partially gratifying instinctual needs without resorting to direct action are many and various. Fantasy is one of the most useful means. The delinquent's capacity for fantasy is often limited. One seldom finds the adolescent delinquent in a relaxed mood, absorbed in spinning a fanciful story. He has a need to plunge indiscriminately into activity. He seems to lack a space in his psychic make-up in which to reflect on ideas. He has no back yard, so to speak. His psyche is all frontage, continuously exposed to new impressions. This one-dimensional psychic structure creates a necessity for the delinquent to act out his impulses and to gain immediate gratification of his needs.

One mechanism used by the mature ego to tolerate frustrations is to invoke the past and recall former gratifications. Most people can recall pleasant experiences and find sufficient satisfaction in them to sustain their spirits during a period of bleakness. The psychic structure of the delinquent apparently is lacking in the ability to retain happy memories. Memories do not have a nourishing value for him. He may speak of a pleasant experience but he does so without emotion. His inability to project himself out of the present affects his relationships not only to the past but to the future.

It has long been recognized that the future has little meaning to the delinquent. He seems to lack capacity to visualize and anticipate experiences in which he will be involved a few weeks or a few days hence. For example, he may engage in a discussion of plans related to school or work, but he does so with a completely blank expression. He may give lip service to the plan, but his comments have a hollow ring. He cannot project himself into the future. Three months hence has as little reality to him as 3000 A.D. does to most people.

The ability to sense the future is one of the ego's most important mechanisms for dealing with reality. The delinquent knows intellectually that there is a future, but his idea of it is vague and devoid of emotional content. He does not comprehend future events with sufficient clarity, or respond to them with sufficient emotion, to influence his behaviour. He is unable to subordinate present desires for future gains. Not being able to recapture the past or to anticipate the future, the delinquent is painfully and tragically dependent on the present. Since he lives in an extreme emotional void, he develops a sense of panic when he is denied immediate gratification of a need. Because of this he is likely to plunge into some questionable activity regardless of the price he may have to pay.

Jerry, a suave, sophisticated-looking 17-year-old boy, manifested extreme panic when his needs were not immediately gratified. He had been placed in a residential treatment centre because of longstanding delinquent behaviour. Whenever any pleasant experience, such as attending a ball game or a movie, was postponed, he became angry; he indulged in profanity and made facial grimaces and hostile gestures. His anger did not seem to be directed specifically towards any one person. Rather it was a diffused reaction of fear and panic set off by his frustration. These feelings created such extreme anxiety that his ego was threatened with disintegration. He lacked a time perspective and had inadequate mechanisms of control.

The narrowness of focus and perception which blurs or sometimes completely obscures the delinquent's sense of the past and the future may also account for the facility with which he gives up relationships, changes loyalties, and shifts plans. He may declare himself in love or he may commit himself irrevocably to a course of action and then make a complete about-face with apparent conflict or guilt. Although such shifts are often attributed to shallowness of feelings or even to conscious fabrication, these explanations are only partially true. During the moments when a delinquent expresses love or determination, he is sincere in his avowal and may have considerable depth and intensity of feeling. When he encounters new situations or new stimuli, however, the past is obliterated and the future is befogged. He reacts only to the present.

If a delinquent is confronted with the fact that he has suddenly changed his opinions, his plan, or his attitude towards a friend, he is likely to respond with a shrug, remarking, 'Isn't a guy allowed to change his mind?' Such sudden shifts indicate that he lacks the capacity to integrate reality. His ego is not able to relate various impressions and experiences to each other and to integrate them. He perceives all experiences—past, present and future—as isolated from each other. They remain separate items in the asset and the debit columns. The ego is unable to relate the plus and minus items to each other and compute a sum total. Thus the delinquent cannot arrive at a unified perception of himself or of others. Lacking in the capacity to integrate reality, he has a fragmented view of the world. To him, good and evil things coexist without interaction. He perceives other people as either all good or all evil. He cannot fuse the two elements in his perception of a person.

The delinquent is often characterized as a person who is unable to learn from experience, as one who repeats an action in spite of his knowledge that it will have negative consequences for him. It has been pointed out that he does not see causality, that his reality testing is impaired, and that his judgement is poor. These generalizations, however, do not stand up under close observation. The delinquent is frequently an astute and shrewd observer of people and their interactions. He is, however, completely unable to observe himself. It is a common experience in an institution to hear a delinquent evaluate realistically the chances of another person's being caught if he engages in a prohibited act. If he speaks of himself, he is sure that he would be able to escape. This feeling of invulnerability stems partly from the sense of omnipotence and the power of magical thinking that are characteristic of the infantile ego. Other psychological processes, however, also account for the delinquent's faulty judgement.

It is my impression that the delinquent utilizes a mechanism which, for lack of a better name, may be called 'selective perception.' The delinquent's ego selects from reality those facts that fit in with his scheme of things and rejects the existence of those that are unpleasant to him or would interfere with his wishes. This process contains elements of avoidance, denial, and negation. Reality to the delinquent has great elasticity. At wish, he can turn it into a hazy dream world. He tends particularly to use the process of selective perception in the area of ethical values. Since the delinquent has a malformed ego structure, his superego is inevitably deficient and distorted—but he *has* the rudiments of a superego. Because the delinquent has a tendency to avoid unpleasant facts, he is able to ignore the prohibitions of the superego if they impinge on his pleasure.

In the course of treatment, Joan, a bright, 20-year-old college girl, frequently cast aspersions at her friends who flirted with married men. Her denunciations were usually accompanied by considerable emotion. For a short period she herself became involved with a married man. Subsequently, after she had progressed in treatment, she talked about this episode and seemed genuinely puzzled about her behaviour. She said, 'I knew he was married but I just put it out of my mind. To me, he was not married. I had no guilt about it.'

The process of selective perception which the delinquent uses to square himself with his superego leads him to distort facts in both crude and subtle ways. His distortions tend to confuse those who endeavour to help him. Often one is unable to follow the delinquent's reversals of feeling and the false links in his association of ideas which lead him to his pseudo-logical conclusions.

The tendency of the delinquent to fragment ideas and experiences is another aspect of the process of selective perception. He detaches one incident from a series of incidents and is unable to perceive the organic relationship between them. He sees an isolated episode instead of the Gestalt. By detaching one incident from the preceding and following ones, he is able to relieve himself of responsibility for his behaviour. For example, a delinquent who extends help to another engaged in a criminal activity is likely to deny his part in the affair or turn it into a virtue, such as loyalty to friends. He does not assume responsibility for his part in the trouble and may argue convincingly that he did not know he was contributing to an illegal act.

Another manifestation of the delinquent's distorted relation to reality is his use of language. In the normal process of development the individual learns to use language as a means of describing reality. The delinquent often retains the infantile trait of equating words with reality. Like a young child, the delinquent attaches magical power to words and believes that they have a potency of their own. Thus he uses words to negate undesirable elements in his reality or to justify his behaviour.

Barbara, a 19-year-old girl, strongly condemned any girl who had a sexual involvement. She referred to her as a 'whore'. However, she appeared to have no scruples about her own sexual activity with her boy friend. She explained that her situation was different because she was in love. She admitted that she had met the boy only recently and that she did not know him very well. By merely naming this relationship 'love' she was able to dissociate her behaviour from the behaviour of the other girls of whom she disapproved. This mechanism made it possible for her to engage in a casual affair even though she had fairly strong superego prohibitions about such behaviour.

The mechanisms that have been discussed above suggest that the individual who handles his internal or external conflicts through delinquent acting-out behaviour suffers from basic ego deficiencies. The delinquent has a core of infantilism in his character structure. My impression is that the nuclear problem of the delinquent lies in faulty ego development and not, as is often suggested, in superego deficiency or superego lacunae. It is the ego of the delinquent that is malformed. It lacks the basic equipment—mechanism of control, capacity for reality testing, ability to bind impulses through language, sublimation, fantasy, and so forth—which is needed to deal with inner and outer stress. Because the delinquent lacks the basic ego tools and has little facility in using those he has, he improvises instruments that almost inevitably lead him to acting-out behaviour.

I should like to offer the following premise: If we scratch a delinquent—regardless of whether his basic dynamics are of a neurotic or social nature—we shall find some malformation of the ego. I believe that the combination of ego deficiency and neurotic guilt leads an individual to resolve his conflict through delinquent behaviour. The individual with an infantile ego does not follow the circuitous route of internalizing impulses and thereby developing neurotic symptoms; he takes the direct route of expressing his impulses openly.

There are, of course, advantages in classifying delinquents according to the essential elements that contribute to their deviant behaviour. When the main impetus and dynamics of the acting-out behaviour is generated by guilt and conflict, the individual may be viewed as a neurotic delinquent. When the chief driving force towards antisocial behaviour is supplied by social and environmental factors, the individual may be classified as a sociological delinquent. When the nuclear problem is an infantile personality, the individual may be classified as a delinquent with a character disorder. The term psychopathic delinquent may sometimes be used for persons with extremely weak superego formation. Not all delinquents fall neatly into one or another of these categories. Often the delinquent presents a combination of psychological problems and deficiencies in emotional development. A diagnostic classification can only suggest the factors that are dominant in propelling an individual into delinquency. I believe that ego deficiency is a thread of varying thickness which runs through all types of delinquent behaviour.

The inconsistencies in the feelings and reactions of a person with a deficient ego are many and varied. He relies on magical power and a sense of omnipotence, but, at the same time, feels extremely helpless and vulnerable. He is capable of engaging in daredevil behaviour and in running extreme risks, but he can also be paralysed by ordinary events that most people take in their stride. He is particularly fearful of physical illnesses or bodily damage. The slightest threat to his body becomes magnified and brings forth anxiety and sometimes panic.

Since I have placed emphasis on the ego malformation of the delinquent and minimized his superego deficiency, I may be asked to justify this emphasis. How can a superego evolve vis-à-vis a poor ego? It is true that the superego is built upon the foundation of the ego, but neither the ego nor the superego is a monolithic structure. Each is a compound of many elements, some of which are present in both. Superego components evolve out of the developed parts of the ego. Hence an individual may attain a level of object relationships and identifications that will permit superego development in certain areas of behaviour. In these areas the superego may be strong enough to generate conflict and guilt. When the infantile ego of the delinquent is confronted with superego prohibitions, it responds by utilizing the same mechanisms it employs to ward off reality dangers. In self-defence the delinquent twists and distorts the injunctions of his superego. He selects and negates facts, uses words magically, and justifies his delinquent activities in various ways. The delinquent has not only a malformed ego but also a fragmented, inconsistent superego. The two interact in subtle and devious ways.

If we accept the premise that ego deficiency is the central cause of delinquent behaviour, we must face certain inevitable questions: What factors are responsible for the deficiency? What treatment techniques can foster further development of the ego? This is not the place to present a formulation of ego development. I can only emphasize the necessity for persons working with delinquents to have an understanding of ego processes, since the central aim of treatment is to enhance ego development.

The treatment techniques for fostering ego development are not as well formulated as the techniques for reducing anxiety and neurotic symptoms. Historically, treatment techniques evolved from work with neurotics, and as a result they are designed to resolve conflicts, reduce guilt, and relax repressive mechanisms. Techniques, therefore, were predicated on the presence of an ego with capacity for object relationships, reality testing, and so forth. It is true that in the neurotic the ego is frequently immobilized by an inhibiting superego but the ego itself has the capacity to perform its functions. In the delinquent, however, basic ego functions have not come into being. The following analogy may clarify the difference. The neurotic is like a person who has well-developed arms that are chained, while the delinquent is like a person whose arms are underdeveloped. If we applied this analogy to treatment, we would say that our objective with the neurotic is to free his ego from its chains while our objective with the delinquent is to stimulate and further the development of his ego.

An essential difference between the treatment approaches to the neurotic and to the delinquent is the nature of the relationship. With the neurotic, one works largely through the transference and deals with the individual's past experiences and internalized images. The therapist utilizes the transference to correct the individual's distorted view of himself and his interpersonal relationships. Since the delinquent lacks the capacity for object relationships, a transference is not easily induced and evolves only gradually. The therapist, in fact, must first endeavour to create a situation that will stimulate the delinquent's capacity to form object relationships and to internalize images. The delinquent must be provided with an experience in the present through which he can master the learning problems of the early development years. He needs a living rather than a reliving experience. The therapist does not represent to the delinquent, as he does to the neurotic, a maternal or a paternal figure. Instead, the therapist functions as a surrogate parent to the delinquent.

Because the therapist must play a parental role, the content of the interviews should be related to the delinquent's immediate concerns and problems. The therapist should endeavour to be helpful in connection with everyday problems no matter how trivial or transitory they may be. He must be available when needed and must be willing to offer guidance and advice. One of the most effective ways to further the relationship with the delinquent is to engage in a discussion of dressing, dating, or sports, or to listen to his gripes. Although such discussion of practical problems have an educational value for the delinquent, their main value lies in the fact that he is drawn into contact with the therapist. By showing concern and by being helpful the therapist plays the role of a parent, and the delinquent, who has strong dependency needs, gradually responds to the helpful and protective parental figure.

As the delinquent responds emotionally, he begins to make some identification with the therapist. Any image of a helpful and protective person which the delinquent will develop will contain the attribute of omnipotence. The primitive, infantile mind can only conceive of helpfulness and protection in terms of omnipotence. This phenomenon creates special problems in treating the delinquent. One problem relates to the handling of the delinquent's image of an omnipotent therapist. In the normal process of growth the young child has little opportunity to test the actual strength and power of his parents. A young boy can have confidence in his picture of his father as a towering Paul Bunyan since he has limited opportunity to check his image against reality. He seldom, if ever, sees his father in a weak position, such as vis-à-vis an employer or other superiors. The physically mature but emotionally infantile delinquent is in a different position. He has a broader perspective and he is more sophisticated. He appraises the therapist by the hierarchic standards of our society and often observes his clay feet. Another complicating factor in handling the delinquent's fantasy of the omnipotence of the therapist is the fact that the therapist actually has some of the powers of control, particularly in an institutional setting, that the delinquent attributes to him.

Because the delinquent is impulsive and volatile, he is consciously and unconsciously preoccupied with the psychological problems of control. He senses that he has tenuous control over his instinctual drives and impulsiveness. He is often impressed with the evenness of temper of the therapist and comments on the fact that he does not get angry or upset. The therapist symbolizes form and order; he is not caught up in the chaotic disorder that dominates the delinquent's world. The therapist's calm is interpreted as omnipotence by the delinquent, and the therapist thus meets the delinquent's need for an omnipotent figure.

In working with the delinquent, the therapist must combine a number of roles that sometimes are considered incompatible. He must be a surrogate parent, a teacher, and a therapist. These various roles gain ascendancy during different phases of treatment, but all may need to be performed concurrently. In a sense, they follow a sequence in treatment. The therapist is first the helpful and protective parent, then a teacher, and finally a clinician who undertakes to help the individual gain some self-understanding.

The therapist must perform a variety of parental functions. In the role of a surrogate parent he must be giving and depriving and must mete out rewards and punishments. He must be all-wise and must be the supreme authority when major issues are involved. These are the attributes in parents that foster ego and superego development in the young child. They create the design of desirable behaviour and the mechanisms for achieving it. The authority exercised by parents in rearing a child has its counterpart in the treatment of a delinquent. In many ways the tasks are analogous, since both the young child and the delinquent have infantile egos which are in the process of developing and taking form.

Analogies, however, may be deceptive. The delinquent and the young child have similarities, but they are not identical. Unlike the child, the delinquent has many years of experience behind him. He has developed certain attitudes towards authority and various mechanisms for dealing with it. He is a master at avoiding and negating any form of authority. In the normal growth process the child learns to accept authority because of his positive feelings towards his parents and his desire to retain their affection. Acceptance of authority is incorporated into the ego and superego structures. The child also develops capacity to observe his own behaviour and to make an objective decision about a course of action. The delinquent, however, did not develop positive feelings towards parental figures in his early years, and consequently he continues to view all forms of authority with suspicion and hostility. Because of his early narcissistic wounds, his feelings of unworthiness, and his fear of retaliation, he is unable to take an objective look at himself. He is extremely sensitive about all personal deficiencies— physical, psychological, and social. He uses extreme denial or rationalization mechanisms to deal with his shortcomings. Unlike the mature individual, he is unable to function simultaneously as an actor and observer.

The dependency of the delinquent is also different from the dependency of the child. The delinquent does not have the same feeling of helplessness, and he does not endow adults with the same protective qualities. Since his base of operation is broader than that of a child, he is not faced with the same limited alternatives—obey or perish.

The early phase of treatment must be characterized by helpfulness on the part of the therapist. He must be a parental figure, but must be a wise, omnipotent, protective parent who is not restrictive and punishing. He must gratify the delinquent's immediate needs and must listen to his hurts and frustrations, but he must not impose rules or set limits. Discussions of social responsibility, values, and ethical standards should not be introduced until later. The delinquent's behaviour, even when it impinges on others, should be discussed only from the vantage point of its repercussions on him. Stealing, for instance, should be discussed in terms of its possible consequences to the thief and not in terms of its effect on others. At no point in treatment, however, should the therapist convey the idea that he condones antisocial behaviour.

The educational process will prove ineffective if it is not continuously merged with, and reinforced by, complementary processes. Educational efforts cannot be introduced until the delinquent has found emotional support in a protective relationship with the therapist; this aspect of treatment, however, gradually becomes dominant. The first step in the educational process is to help the delinquent see the patterns of his behaviour. Often the therapist must confront him with these patterns. Because the delinquent is absorbed in the present and is constantly acting out his impulses, he has little awareness of the nature of his behaviour or of the reaction of others towards it. The therapist begins by pointing out to the delinquent that he repeats certain actions and that they inevitably lead to certain consequences. In time the delinquent is able to combine isolated incidents and begin to identify a pattern of behaviour. He then is gradually able to recognize some of the mechanisms he employs, such as his tendency to avoid painful experiences and to dissociate himself from responsibility for his behaviour.

Gradually, as the delinquent gains the capacity to observe himself, he becomes more anxious and, often, more introspective. He is usually then able to explore the origins of his mechanisms. This phase of treatment is similar to the treatment of the neurotic, but it is different in the sense that the therapist must continue to play the roles of surrogate parent and teacher. The therapist must guard against the risk of instituting introspective techniques too soon or at inappropriate times. The wrong approach is likely to set back treatment and, in some instances, to undermine the relationship completely.

In this brief discussion of treatment techniques, I have been able only to outline a general approach. The outline suggests an orderliness of procedures that does not prevail in actual practice. I have mentioned that the therapist must play three roles in treating the delinquent, and that successful treatment progresses through three stages. It should not be assumed that these stages occur in a clear-cut sequence; in reality they overlap and swing back and forth. The three roles played by the therapist continue throughout the course of treatment, although one may be more prominent than the others at certain points.

11

A CONCEPT OF ACUTE
SITUATIONAL DISORDERS*

DAVID M. KAPLAN

IN recent years a number of social workers have made a plea for further study and clarification of current conceptualization of casework problems, out of a sense of dissatisfaction with these concepts and the related system of classifying casework problems.[1] The importance of these formulations of casework problems to diagnosis, to treatment, and to the growing professional interest in developing preventive measures makes the task of clarifying these concepts one of high priority. This paper is offered in the hope that it may contribute a new theoretical framework from which to view the definitions and classification of casework problems.

There is consensus that a casework problem involves an individual who is out of harmony with his environment; an individual who has failed to reach a satisfactory adjustment between his desires and his conditions of life. Although there are certain variations in the ways in which social workers have defined and classified casework problems, there is agreement that these problems fall into two major categories: (1) Environmental and (2) Individual.[2]

This dichotomous classification has important implications for practice in that *each problem category prescribes what is considered to be*

* Published in *Social Work*, New York, Vol. VII, No. 2, April, 1962.

[1] Henry S. Maas, 'Psychiatric Clinic Services for Children: 1. Unanswered Questions', *Social Service Review*, Vol. XXX, No. 2, September, 1956, pp. 276–88; Werner W. Boehm, *The Social Casework Method in Social Work Education*, Vol. X of the Curriculum Study Council on Social Work Education, New York, 1959, pp. 30–2; Dorothy F. Beck, 'Research Relevant to Casework Treatment of Children: Current Research and Study Projects', *Social Casework*, Vol. XXXIX, Nos. 2–3, February–March, 1958, pp. 106–7.

[2] See Boehm, op. cit., p. 20; Beck, op. cit., p. 107; Lilian Ripple, 'Motivation, Capacity and Opportunity as Related to the Use of Casework Service: Theoretical Base and Plan of Study', *Social Service Review*, Vol. XX, No. 2, June, 1955, p. 187; Helen H. Perlman, 'Social Casework', *Social Work Year Book 1960*, National Association of Social Workers, New York, 1960, pp. 535–40; Florence Hollis, 'Social Casework', *Social Work Year Book 1957*, National Association of Social Workers, New York, 1957, pp. 527–8.

the remedial core of that problem. The problem category indicates whether casework efforts of modification should be directed towards the environment or towards the individual to resolve the problem.

Environmental problems include those maladjustments in which unfavourable changes in environmental conditions precipitate the problem for the individual. The unfavourable environmental conditions that bring about an environmental problem occur in the course of normal living and not as a consequence of existing pathology within the individual. Economic depressions, wars, deaths, and serious illnesses are examples of unfavourable conditions which precipitate environmental problems for individuals.

In addition to their extrapathologic origin, environmental problems are defined, implicitly, as problems with intrapsychic consequences only when the precipitating conditions are allowed to continue uncorrected. Therefore, remedial casework efforts in regard to environmental problems are directed primarily towards changing unfavourable environmental conditions to more favourable ones. This casework goal is accomplished either by (1) offering services to meet 'unmet needs' or by (2) removing harmful external pressures that impinge on the individual.[1] As the term suggests, an environmental problem is theoretically a problem that can be corrected by modifying the individual's environment. When such modifications are successful, the individual emerges from this situation presumably without damage to his psychic structure.

Individual problems, in contrast to environmental difficulties, are considered to develop as a result of intrapsychic maladjustments which are an inherent and persisting part of the individual's personality.[2] As such they are less likely to respond to favourable changes in environmental conditions. Basic to this problem conceptualization is the presence in the individual of an established and continuing disease process, a necessary condition for this type of problem. Casework efforts in relation to individual problems are therefore directed towards effecting changes 'within the individual', either by (1) supportive treatment or by (2) developing self-awareness.[3]

If one accepts the idea that the problems which casework seeks to resolve are largely the result of life experiences, it is clear that individual problems are derivative—i.e. a consequence of the unsuccessful resolution of environmental difficulties. A problem becomes internalized when the individual fails to make a satisfactory adjustment to one or

---

[1] Hollis, op. cit., p. 527.
[2] Perlman, op. cit., p. 535.
[3] Hollis, loc. cit.

more problems while they are still considered to be environmental. For this reason casework has a considerable stake in the successful mastery of environmental problems to fulfil the professional goals of promoting healthy development of the individual and his capacity for effective functioning, and preventing disease processes of long duration from becoming established.

Despite the importance of successfully resolving environmental problems, there is a tendency among caseworkers, which Werner Boehm has noted, to devalue casework directed towards the solution of environmental problems.[1] A part of this attitude seems to be attributable to the way in which these problems have been defined. The current conception of environmental problems appears to exclude the possibility that *distinctive and significant psychological processes* are involved in the early reaction of the individual to the environmental conditions that precipitate these problems.

In casework practice, consideration is given to the psychological processes that accompany environmental problems, but these processes are commonly perceived as being essentially the same as those recognized in individual problems. But while individual responses to environmental problems do involve familiar psychological phenomena, there is evidence to suggest that these processes are organized and structured in a unique fashion when observed in relation to environmental problems.

Also absent from the environmental problem conception is the possibility that such internal processes may play a significant role in determining whether intrapsychic damage results, *irrespective of casework modifications of the precipitating conditions.* These conclusions seem to be warranted by the absence of any reference to the role of relevant internal processes in the description of environmental problems, and by the clear statement that these problems can be resolved primarily by modification of environmental conditions.[2]

Under the terms of the present definition, environmental problems are strangely devoid of any human or personal response to the unfavourable conditions that bring them about. Environmental problems, as currently defined, consist of external conditions that are not meaningfully related to the human beings who experience and respond to them. The definition in its present form is comparable to describing an equation by referring only to one of its sides. Is it surprising, then, that caseworkers have less interest in environmental than in individual

[1] Boehm, op. cit., p. 30.
[2] Hollis, loc. cit.

problems—the latter being defined largely in terms of human response and reaction to life experiences?

Florence Hollis has observed that the two major forms of casework treatment, environmental and individual, are often combined in casework practice.[1] This is certainly true, but it does not follow therefrom that environmental problems are perceived as having their own distinctive internal aspects. The fact that casework practice often involves both types of treatment does not mean that individual treatment, as currently conceived and constituted, can deal effectively with the internal reactions that occur as a result of environmental problems.

It is possible to explain the combination of both types of casework treatment in practice by the fact that individuals often confront environmental and individual problems simultaneously. However, if environmental problems have their own distinctive internal aspects— which is the present writer's contention—it is important to distinguish the type(s) of problem faced (environmental or individual or both) and then bring to bear the appropriate casework skills that are required to resolve the problem(s) involved. The fact that individual treatment techniques may also be used in casework with an individual confronted by an environmental problem does not offer assurance that these techniques are adequate to resolve the distinctive internal aspects of any and all environmental problems.

Helen Perlman makes essentially the same point in differentiating 'basic problems' from 'problems-to-be-solved.'[2] A 'problem-to-be-solved', she notes, is often superimposed upon a 'basic problem', but the close proximity should not conceal from us that two different kinds of problems are involved, and that each calls for its own treatment techniques. An individual who has a chronic heart condition may also contract pneumonia; to treat him successfully it is necessary to recognize that he has two separate problems, each of which has its own unique characteristics requiring distinctive treatment.[3] Quite possibly the same principle applies in dealing with casework problems.

Recently a number of studies have been made of human problems precipitated by specific upsetting events.[4] These unbalancing events are either the product of circumstances beyond individual control (e.g.

[1] Hollis, loc. cit.
[2] Helen H. Perlman, *Social Casework: A Problem-Solving Process*, Chicago: University of Chicago Press, 1957, p. 32.
[3] While each disease process requires its own treatment it is also true that the presence of two concurrent disorders will modify the total treatment plan.
[4] Erich Lindemann, 'Symtomatology and Management of Acute Grief', *American Journal of Psychiatry*, Vol. CI, No. 2, September, 1944; I. L. Janis, *Psychological Stress*, John Wiley & Sons, New York, 1958; Kaplan, op. cit.

disasters and economic dislocations) or occur in the course of normal living (e.g. illnesses and deaths); but they do not stem from the existing psychopathology of the individuals involved. From these studies a clearer perception is emerging of the inner psychological processes involved in the individual's struggle to master unfavourable environmental conditions. These studies and the theoretical formulations derived from them suggest that the process of adaptation in an individual faced with stress-producing conditions involves distinctive organizations of intrapsychic phenomena which are essential for caseworkers to understand if they are to play a more meaningful role in the resolution of this group of human problems.

Erich Lindemann, in his study of bereavement reactions, was one o1 the first investigators to describe the existence and significance of the psychological processes involved in environmental problems.[1] From his observation of the survivors and relatives of the victims of the Cocoanut Grove fire in Boston, Lindemann discovered that this group suffered from a well-defined psychological disturbance which was a direct reaction to the bereavement involved. The clinical picture he observed resembled that commonly seen in depressive types of psychiatric illness, but in the majority of cases the clinical syndrome proceeded through certain characteristic phases and disappeared in four to six weeks. Lindemann referred to the successful adaptive responses to bereavement as 'courses of normal grief reaction'. In a number of cases frank psychiatric and psychosomatic illnesses developed. Lindemann referred to these maladaptive responses as 'morbid grief reactions'.

Lindemann learned that successful mastery of the problem posed by the loss of a loved person was accomplished through 'grief work', a process of specific adaptive behaviour first described by Freud, in which the bereaved person seeks to extricate himself from bondage to the deceased and to find new paths of rewarding interaction.[2] As a result of his work, Lindemann concluded that:

'At first glance acute grief would not seem to be a clinical or psychiatric disorder in the strict sense of the word, but rather a normal reaction to a distressing situation. However, the understanding of reactions to traumatic experiences whether or not they represent clear-cut neuroses has become of ever-increasing importance to the psychiatrist. Bereavement or sudden cessation of social interaction seemed to be of special

[1] Lindemann, op. cit.
[2] S. Freud, 'Mourning and Melancholia', *Collected Papers*, Vol. V, Hogarth Press, London, 1925, pp. 152–70.

interest because it is often cited among the alleged psychogenic factors in psychosomatic disorders.'[1]

Gerald Caplan, in summarizing the implications of Lindemann's study of reactions in acute grief situations, observed that (1) Lindemann's research described the complete range of individual responses to loss by death from the adaptive to the maladaptive. (2) Such reactions were typically limited in time from four to six weeks. The symptoms observed were not signs of psychiatric illness but the 'epiphenomena of the adaptive process'. (3) Intervention in such crises was directed primarily towards helping the bereaved person to go through with the grieving process and not to analysing why people could not grieve unaided. (4) Intervention in this situation did not have to be undertaken by psychiatrists, whose skills were properly reserved for etiological analysis.[2]

Lindemann's study of bereavement reactions suggests that in the course of everyday living there occur a wide variety of events that precipitate acute dislocations for the individual. These dislocations are reflected in lowered levels of social functioning and higher levels of anxiety and personal distress. For the most part the problems created by such disequilibrating events have not received the clinical attention or importance they deserve, although they are so often forerunners of serious chronic problems.

Disequilibrating events, such as death, *create new situations for the individual*—a new set of circumstances to which he is required to make an adjustment. Whether the individual's adaptation is healthy or not, whether he masters the new situation or fails to do so, the *adaptation occurs in a given social setting and in a given period of time initiated by the dislocating event.*

The concept of 'situation' as an aspect of human problems is not a new idea in casework. Ada E. Sheffield in 1937 argued that *the individual confronted with a problem situation* was the appropriate 'unit of attention' in casework because the concept of 'situation' designates the treatment unit as a 'segment of experience' and not the individual alone. Sheffield wrote, '... when social casework is most intelligent and thorough, the worker does deal with situations rather than with individuals or even with families'.[3] The importance attached to the 'situation' as a

[1] Lindemann, op. cit., p. 141.
[2] G. Caplan, 'An Approach to the Study of Family Mental Health', *Public Health Reports*, Vol. LXXI, No. 10, October, 1956, pp. 1027-30.
[3] Ada E. Sheffield, *Social Insight in Case Situations*, D. Appleton-Century Company, New York, 1937, p. 79.

factor to be considered in casework practice and teaching has varied over the years, but the value of understanding and meeting the individual in the context of the situation he perceives and is concerned with has long been recognized as sound casework practice.

While there has been recognition for some time that certain commonly recurring events have important psychological and situational components, Lindemann's unique contribution has been to provide a theoretical framework by which these events and the human responses to them (adaptive and maladaptive) can be conceptualized, studied and treated. The studies that have been made of bereavement, of combat fatigue reactions, and of responses to surgery and to premature birth suggest the existence of a category of *acute situational problems*. This group of problems has features in common with Perlman's category of 'problems-to-be-solved' and with Dorothy A. Beck's suggested classification of 'crisis problems'. A large number of problems now referred to as environmental appear to be examples of acute situational problems.

Acute situational problems occur when three conditions have been met. The *first condition* is the existence of the relevant non-pathological characteristic(s) in an individual without which the problem cannot occur; fertility, for birth problems; appropriate age for retirement problems; racial traits for problems of discrimination; and so on. The *second condition* consists of those values inherent in the individual by virtue of which an event is perceived as a personal threat: thus premature birth is a problem for a mother when she values carrying the pregnancy through to term; retirement constitutes a threat to an individual when he places a high value on his position as an active, productive person and perceives retirement as involving a loss of this position. The internalized individual values generally reflect the values of the culture and the subculture to which he belongs. The *third condition* consists of occurrence of events that constitute a threat to the individual: premature birth, death in the family, diagnosis of a chronic illness, and so on.

The first condition (existence of relevant individual characteristics) and the second (existence of relevant values) define the *susceptible population* for a particular situational problem. When these conditions have been met, the third condition (occurrence of the threatening event) determines the *group of casualties* that will occur for any situational problem.

Casework problem conceptualizations contain, explicitly or implicitly, some reference to the state of health of the individual involved.

In current casework problem classification the concept of disease used is based upon psychoanalytic theory and analytic nosology. Lindemann, in his study of grief reactions, made implicit use of a concept of disease derived, not from traditional psychiatric nosology, but from the disease theory of somatic medicine. He adopted the disease theory employed in medicine to diagnose and treat acute infectious diseases, with appropriate modifications to make it applicable to behavioural phenomena. The close basic and parallel similarity of the theoretical model underlying the acute infectious diseases and the model used to study situational problems suggests another order of psychological disturbances, that of *acute situational disturbances due to the occurrence of threatening events, where the disturbances are not simply exacerbations of chronic diseases.*

From the viewpoint of nosological classification, it is possible to conceive of two distinct classes among emotional disorders, analogs of similar classes recognized in somatic disorders—namely, chronic and acute disturbances. The personality or characterological problem of psychiatry is essentially the chronic emotion disorder, e.g. the neurosis, psychosis, character disorder. These psychological disorders are analogous to the complex somatic diseases—heart disease, cancer, arthritis, and the like. Whether they are of psychological or somatic origin, chronic disorders have certain characteristics in common. They invariably refer to internalized or structural defects that persist over relatively long periods of time. They are generally not self-correcting. Their etiologies are a result of many complexly interwoven determinants, whose origins often go back for years in the history of the individual. The treatment of chronic disorders usually requires considerable expenditure of effort over long periods of time to achieve ameliorative success of any consequence.

There are essentially two types of acute disturbances. One refers to acute problems that stem from previously existing chronic conditions—for instance, a flare-up of tuberculosis in a previously quiescent case. An acute psychotic episode arising out of an established schizophrenia is an example of the same type of acute exacerbation in the field of psychological disorders.

The second type of acute disorder is exemplified by the acute infectious diseases. Many childhood diseases fall into this category, such as measles, chicken pox, polio, and so on. The occurrence of such a disorder does not depend upon the prior existence of an established chronic process but *results from the individual's attempt to cope with an external force for which he does not have adequate defences at the onset of the disorder. The absence of such defences does not imply structural defects, for the necessary defensive forces can be produced after the onset of the disease.*

Acute infectious disorders are casually related to identifiable 'etiologic agents', on the one hand, and to the level of bodily defences available to deal with these agents on the other. An acute infectious disorder does not occur unless the etiologic agent succeeds in invading a susceptible host. When acute infectious disorders do occur, outcome from them is variable; the noxious agents may be successfully walled off and destroyed, or they may be unsuccessfully dealt with, leading to complications and sequelae. It has been proved possible to intervene during the course of acute disorders by strengthening the resisting defensive forces of the host, reducing thereby the severity and harmful effect of such disorders.

In the field of psychological disorders, we do not currently have a conception of acute emotional disorders of the nonchronic type which approximates that of the acute somatic model. During World War Two a number of psychiatrists utilized an acute disease model to treat emotional combat casualties.[1] Interestingly enough, however, the acute disease model was rejected theoretically when the 'war neuroses' were classified as merely one form of 'true neurosis' and not as a separate disease phenomenon or as a separate nosological category.[2]

Current psychiatric nosology is almost entirely one of chronic disorders. Lawrence Kubie describes the nature of illness amenable to psychiatric treatment as follows:

'The ills which are subjected to psychoanalytic treatment are never acute or passing ailments. For the most part they are chronic illnesses with occasional periods of acute exacerbation. The quiescent chronic phases of neurotic illness may often be mistaken for normality, just as the sufferer from tuberculosis may seem to be normal in the intervals between attacks for years before his infection first manifests itself openly. As Glover pointed out, there are illuminating analogies between the problems of treatment in the two illnesses. In each, the acute episodes may be of short duration; but the physician who is willing to discharge a patient as cured immediately after such an

---

[1] K. Goldstein, 'On So-called War Neuroses', *Psychosomatic Medicine*, Vol. V, No. 4, October, 1943; H. N. Raines and L. C. Kolb, 'Combat Fatigue and War Neuroses', *U.S. Naval Medicine Bulletin*, Vol. XLI, No. 4, July, 1943; S. Rado, 'Pathodynamics and Treatment of Traumatic War Neuroses', *Psychosomatic Medicine*, Vol. IV, No. 4, October, 1942.

[2] R. Grinker and J. P. Spiegel, *Men Under Stress*, Blakiston Co., Philadelphia, 1945, p. 348.

episode is either incompetent or unscrupulous. It is only when a sufferer from tuberculosis has become temporarily symptom-free that the long march towards enduring health begins. The same principle is valid in the treatment of neurosis. It is unreasonable to think that lifelong illnesses, be they low grade chronic infections, or marked neurotic traits, can be cured in a short time. In both, one measures the duration of adequate treatment in terms of years and not of months.'[1]

An acute emotional disorder need not depend conceptually or actually upon the prior existence of an established chronic disease any more than acute infectious disorder does. *Such a disorder can result from the individual's attempt to cope with a threatening psychological event for which he is not sufficiently prepared at the outset.*

This concept of situationally initiated illness does not preclude the fact that a proportion of the reactions to a stressful event will be heavily conditioned by previously existing personality factors or chronic conditions. However, even when such chronic conditions exist they do not necessarily determine outcome. Chronic illnesses are neither necessary nor sufficient conditions for the occurrence of acute disorders. There are current environmental forces which have an important bearing on outcome, because the reaction to an acute problem is a manifestation of defensive struggle in which the outcome is at issue and therefore dependent on the adequacy of the defensive forces the individual musters to overcome the problem.

There are certain important parallels between the individual's psychological reaction to a stressful event and the physiological reaction of an individual to a disease-producing agent. In acute psychological disorders *the counterpart of the 'etiologic agent' of acute infectious diseases is the threatening event which disequilibrates the individual* and to which he struggles to make an adaptation. Most responses to situational stress regardless of outcome are self-correcting; the individual regains some form of equilibrium on his own. The severity of reactions to a psychologically stressful event varies from the mild to the severe as the severity of responses to an infectious organism does. The individual subjected to such events experiences stress in the form of painful subjective symptoms. In addition, his social functioning is affected, at least temporarily. The symptoms that occur, though they may resemble the signs of frank psychiatric disorders, are rather signs of a temporary disequilibrium and usually disappear when a new equilibrium is restored.

[1] L. Kubie, *Practical and Theoretical Aspects of Psychoanalysis*, International Universities Press, New York, 1950, p. 39.

The individual whose psychic balance has been so upset strives to regain a state of equilibrium by mastering the problems that the event poses for him. The struggle for mastery is relatively brief, culminating in some form of resolution of the problem. The resolution may be healthy or unhealthy, depending upon how the problem is dealt with, but—regardless of outcome—the disequilibrium is generally brief and self-correcting. When the resolution is unhealthy, there are specifiable sequelae and/or complications that affect role functioning and personality subsequent to the acute disturbance.

Because the threatening event, which corresponds to the etiologic agent of infectious diseases, is specific and fixed in time, the focus of such a problem is highly circumscribed. The psychological tasks that must be accomplished in order successfully to master a situational problem can be clearly specified. The range of responses, both adaptive and maladaptive, is not infinite or highly idiosyncratic but can be described in a limited number of 'courses' leading either to healthy or unhealthy outcome. *Healthy outcome is the result of adaptive responses* that enable the individual to accomplish the tasks posed by the problem. *Unhealthy outcome is a result of maladaptive responses* that do not enable the individual to deal adequately with them.

Because the concept of the cause of disease in the acute infectious model is twofold, involving the interaction of defensive factors in the individual on the one hand and noxious forces in the environment on the other, it has proved possible to protect the healthy in a community from ever contracting certain of these diseases. This result has been achieved by preventing the disease-producing factors of the environment from invading the susceptible host—e.g. by separating sewage from water supplies. When it is not possible to keep the host free from infection, it is often possible to strengthen the individual by immunization or by therapeutic measures so that the infection either does not cause clinically recognizable forms of disease or is modified and weakened considerably in its effect.

What are some of the implications of the acute situational problem concept for casework problem typology? The concept of acute situational problems presupposes that there are distinguishable patterns and distinctive internal processes involved in individual responses to unfavourable environmental conditions. In effect, this problem conception adds a new dimension to the environmental problem conception—the dimension of an *individual psychological reaction to environmental conditions* which is of critical importance in the resolution of these problems.

The situational problem conception suggests that casework problems are not really divided into problems that are external on the one hand or internal on the other; it supports the idea that all casework problems have a significant internal aspect. A truer division of casework problems may be related to the type of underlying disorder involved. *Individual* problems are those in which the presence of a chronic psychological disorder is a necessary condition. *Situational* problems involve adaptive reactions to changes in environmental conditions, in which disturbance of the individual is acute and presence of a chronic disorder is not a necessary condition for the existence of the problem.

The situational problem concept has certain implications for casework practice. Because the acute situational problem concept of cause is framed in terms of factors within both the individual and the environment, both types of factors have significance in the resolution and treatment of this type of problem, as they have significance for the etiology of this disturbance. The diagnosis and treatment of acute situational problems are focused, therefore, not only on the individual and his problem-solving efforts, but on all environmental factors that can affect his adaptive response, whether favourably or adversely. The behaviour of community agency representatives—indeed, the policies of these agencies—may be highly relevant to the resolution of the problem with which the individual is struggling. The behaviour of close family members during this struggle may have critical significance for outcome as well.

It is of considerable importance for those involved in the treatment of individuals facing situational problems, therefore, to have firsthand knowledge of how the behaviour of community personnel and family members may affect the individual in his problem-solving efforts. In premature birth, for example, the behaviour of hospital personnel who come in contact with the mother can help or seriously hinder the mother's problem-solving responses, just as the husband's behaviour can aid or impede the mother in her attempts to cope with the fact that she has given birth to a premature infant. The sound treatment of acute situational problems requires intervention directed towards the behaviour of significant persons involved in the problem as much as towards the mother herself, when help is indicated.[1]

The diagnosis and treatment of acute situational problems take into account the ego-adaptive responses of the individual specified in

[1] D. M. Kaplan and E. A. Mason, 'Maternal Reactions to Premature Birth Viewed as an Acute Emotional Disorder', *American Journal of Orthopsychiatry*, Vol. XXX, No. 3, July, 1960, pp. 539–47.

identifiable 'courses' of response; also etiological diagnoses of personality, to the extent that such diagnoses are significant for differential treatment. Courses of response leading to healthy and unhealthy outcome permit prognoses to be made which separate individuals dealing successfully with the problem from those who do not. Such prognoses serve to protect individuals in difficulty by allowing treatment resources to be brought to their aid. They also make possible more economical use of resources by eliminating from treatment persons who are solving their problems adequately on their own. Because acute reactions have clearly definable onsets and brief periods of duration, treatment can be limited to this definable, brief period of time. The adaptive psychological tasks in a situational problem can be defined with considerable specificity, and the treatment of such problems can be specifically defined to a comparable degree.[1]

The concept of acute situational disorders may conceivably also have important preventive implications for casework problems. Such a concept in the field of behavioural phenomena could serve to protect the healthy population in a community and to prevent the development of chronic disorders, either by precluding certain threatening events from impinging on susceptible individuals or by bolstering individual resources, so that when these events occur they need not have so destructive an effect. For example, as a community eliminates unemployment by economic measures, it effectively removes the threat that unemployment poses for individuals in the working population. Social and unemployment insurance programmes are methods of reducing the traumatic effect of income loss occasioned by unemployment. Before the existence of these programmes, unemployment created individual crises of considerably greater magnitude, and job loss constituted a situation involving considerably higher mental health risk.

[1] Ibid.

12

INTERPRETING REJECTION
TO ADOPTIVE APPLICANTS*

ALFRED L. KASPROWICZ

THE question of whether to discuss with adoptive applicants the reasons for their rejection is fraught with controversy. The trend seems to be to tell the prospective parents the reason for rejection in a face-to-face interview rather than in a general non acceptance letter, yet there remains much reserve and hesitation on the part of the worker in putting these ideas into practice. This resistance causes one to wonder if adoption workers really approve of this procedure.

When workers are questioned about why they do not follow through more thoroughly in explaining to clients the reasons for their rejection, their responses are quite similar—they all imply a fear of harming the existing family relationships. The most common reason given is to avoid telling a couple anything that might disturb or weaken the marriage. If the cause of rejection is the behaviour of a child already in the family, the worker may fear that the parents will project the blame for their rejection upon the child. Another fear expressed by some caseworkers is that the couple will not be able to cope with the anxiety created by a focus on their deficiencies. Many workers wonder if working through with the couple the anxiety thus produced is a legitimate function of an adoption agency. If so, in view of the pressing backlog of cases in most adoption agencies, can the worker afford the time needed to resolve these conflicts? These are the reasons given, but behind these lie several more. It is possible that the worker fears handling difficult situations or that he is not sure of his findings; refusing to discuss them is the easy way out.

There is much to be gained by telling the couple why their application is being rejected. The effects of not giving adoptive applicants sufficient information about their rejection are varied and troublesome.

* Published in *Social Work*, New York, Vol. IX, No. 1, January, 1964.

The writer knows of no adoption agency that has not experienced the pressure and threat of a disappointed couple who want to know why they were rejected. Although disappointed clients will continue to exist, the amount of antagonism and hostility towards the worker and the agency will decrease markedly if the reasons for their non acceptance are dealt with in a direct, competent, and professional manner.

To see the adoptive situation in its proper perspective, workers must imagine themselves in the role of the applicant. They must be aware of the applicants' attitudes about an agency before they come to it. It is common knowledge that prospective adoptive couples have many misgivings about going to an agency in view of all they have heard. Adoption agencies must accept the fact that their images in the minds of many adoptive couples and, for that matter, in the minds of a wide segment of the community, are based on newspaper publicity and accounts of how they have wrenched unfortunate children from the arms of sweet, warm, and generous adoptive parents. To the public, then, the behaviour of a professional social agency often appears to be contrary to common sense, good judgement, and reason. Consequently, the anxious adoptive couple, having heard vicious rumours, are all the more determined to be on their guard while still trying to be as co-operative as possible on the surface.

It is partly to clear up false impressions that many adoption agencies hold orientation meetings. These sessions have three basic objectives: (1) to correct the erroneous beliefs and misconceptions of applicants, (2) to give them the correct information about the agency and its procedures, (3) to use the group meeting as a method of observing the couples' group interaction as a beginning for diagnostic thinking.

While group meetings may correct many false impressions and alleviate some fears, many areas of concern cannot be adequately handled by this process. In the first place, the very nature of the couple's inability to have children may create an aura of inadequacy that cannot be entirely dispelled through a group meeting. Couples wonder if their sterility has been predestined by God. The anxious and insecure woman may damage her self-image even further by the uneasy, unconscious feelings of inadequacy because of her infertility. The writer's observation is that infertility in a woman has greater psychological ramifications for her than it does for a man. To the man, it may interfere with a comfortable feeling in regard to his masculinity but may not necessarily impair his image of successful fatherhood. On the other hand, infertility in a woman can often create doubt as to her capacity to fulfil the demands of motherhood. She may wonder if she has what it takes really to love a child and to be a whole woman. Thus, it is not uncommon for a woman who feels uncertain about her capacity for motherhood to become overprotective after the placement of the first child, but this can also be found in a natural parent. The natural mother has the opportunity to reach the psychological zenith of motherhood whereas the adoptive mother must wait in anxious anticipation and, while waiting, create even greater problems of anxiety and self-doubt.

In addition to the insecurity resulting from their inability to have children and from their fear of an agency itself, couples are often painfully aware of their own personality defects. They may fear that the social worker will find out how they really feel about themselves. In other cases, although the couple may not be consciously aware of any inadequacies, they may still be anxious about what hidden personality defects may be uncovered by the social worker.

Just as social workers as individuals have developed compensatory defences for their deficiencies, so have adoptive clients. More time ought to be spent studying clients' ego defences as indicated in their social histories in addition to finding out the traumatic and damaging aspects of their early childhood. Just as social workers have their own blind spots about faults in their personality structures, so do adoptive parents. Workers become defensive and want proof and examples of where they have failed in fulfilling their duties when confronted with this by their supervisors; so do the adoptive parents. Workers feel better when they can rationalize and pull their defensive structure together when challenged with threatening information; so do they. And just as a supervisor hopes for some insight on behalf of the worker by sharing his observations, workers desire the same of their adoptive clients.

Adoptive clients deeply appreciate the worker's willingness to give them the opportunity of defending themselves when presented with the reasons for rejection. Although they will attack or cry, deny or admit, get angry or become defensive, and even scream during the process, they will often come away from an interview with a better feeling about the agency. Most important, they have been provided with an opportunity to discuss their weaknesses, to understand themselves better, and to seek help if this is indicated.

There are, of course, dangers to this approach. Interpretation of the dynamics of personality is not something that should be taken lightly, nor should it be undertaken by those who have no training or awareness of this process. An interpretation should never be given hastily.

It requires adequate time and preparation and a thorough knowledge of the couple's dynamics.

The manner in which interpretation is done is important. There is an inherent reluctance on the part of most persons to hurt another individual. Workers are aware that the interpretation of unpleasant material may be painful to clients and, to lessen the unconscious feelings of their guilt, some of them tend to detach themselves from the interpretive process and to handle the rejection in a cold, impersonal way. Without a doubt this manner of interpretation arouses hostility on the part of the client. Moreover, the worker does not have the right to shatter a person's defences without being concerned over what defences will take their place. In contrast to the results of a cold, impersonal approach, a warm and sympathetic interpretation will provide for a direct continuation of the helping process of casework. Proper use of this technique requires skill and training, but the development of this skill is not beyond the capabilities of most workers.

Basically, if the worker follows three general principles he may discover that the interpretive session need not be difficult. Briefly stated, these rules are: (1) interpret only the material obtained from clients in the course of the interviews, (2) get all the facts from a well-prepared social history, (3) discuss problem areas with the clients as they arise rather than spring rejection on them as a surprise.

The whole concept of interpreting dynamics to another individual is clouded with confusion. The popular misconception is that interpretation implies interpreting deeply from the unconscious. Although this may be so in an intense analytical session, it is doubtful whether it is a true definition of what is generally meant by most people who use this technique. The consensus seems to be that in order for interpretation to be effective, one can only interpret material that the client has brought out in the interviews. Although one can interpret one's own intuitions and hunches, these 'guesses' must have their basis in the material verbally elicited from the client or in the interaction experienced with him. To state it more simply, the social worker cannot interpret his inferences unless the client has verbally expressed or discussed material leading to these inferences. To do otherwise allows the client to reject the interpretation, deny its validity, or become extremely anxious.

In many adoption agencies it is the procedure to hold a conference or 'staffing' on an especially difficult case. The format is essentially the same in all agencies. The social worker presents findings based upon the social history and his interviews with the client. The purpose of the other participants is to see what additional insight they can bring out in order to establish a better diagnostic understanding of the couple's personalities. In the diagnostic process it is not unusual for one member to make interpretations based on someone else's inference. This kind of interpretation is dangerous, especially if the worker is left with cumulative results of these interpretations based upon the inferences of others. Such conclusions create a tremendous problem for the worker who is left with the job of handling the results of the discussion with the client. The difficulty the worker faces in rejecting the adoptive couple's application is not so much found in the diagnosed pathology as in how he is to handle this material with his clients. The question remains, 'How can the worker share with the client diagnostic material that has been gained through inference?' The natural outcome is that the worker will seek to avoid the uncomfortable situation and will structure an appropriate rationale for doing so.

This difficult situation can be remedied most of the time if the worker makes sure that he gets the necessary data on which to base a judgement. Many of the problems encountered in interpreting sessions with clients stem from an inadequate or incomplete social history. One of the problems in interviewing appears to be that workers fail to go far enough in soliciting data. In a review of the clients' early background they obtain necessary background data and then fail to take the additional step of soliciting the client's reaction to the data. By neglecting to do this the workers are left with the facts but no knowledge of what these facts mean to the client. For example, it is not enough to know that the client's parents were strict or punitive; the effect the client feels this had upon him must also be known. This conclusion cannot be drawn from inference no matter how logical it may appear. Although experience and knowledge of the universals of behaviour help the worker to fill many of the gaps, he cannot substitute his own conclusions for the feelings of the client.

All workers have experienced situations in which their judgements were wrong. From a set of facts a legitimate inference may be made; yet, upon the client being asked what effect this set of circumstances had upon him, it is often surprising to learn that he does not always come to the same conclusions. The fact that the client does not concur with the worker's inference does not always mean that the worker had judged incorrectly; actually, his drawing a different conclusion from a given set of facts may be a good lead and diagnostic clue. It may be indicative of the client's blocking or resistance to a problem area that needs to be pursued further. Thus, this type of interviewing skill and the obtaining of information cannot be left to chance but must become a basic part of the social worker's interviewing ability.

It is also vital for the worker to inform the adoptive applicants at the outset that he may come across information that may cause him concern, and if he does, he will discuss it with them frankly. Such an approach, instead of creating anxiety, actually reduces it. Clients are aware that they have problems. The fact that they may have consciously avoided discussing a problem creates more anxiety because of their fear of being found out. Yet if they know in advance that the worker will discuss his questions, at least they have the feeling that when the time comes to open up their particular difficulties they will have a chance to justify themselves. This positive kind of attitude is far superior to that of the client who does not know what the worker is thinking or how he is being judged.

Thus, the thesis of this article is that *unless the worker has sufficiently discussed and explored the couple's difficulties in the social history session, he is not in a position to discuss reasons for rejecting them.* The situation is analogous to a worker who, when he receives his evaluation from his supervisor, encounters all sorts of critical observations for the first time, many of which may be valid but which have never been brought up before. He immediately wants the supervisor to prove his observations or to substantiate them in some way. When this happens, the supervisor is generally uncomfortable, has to fall back on the authority of his position, or may have to present weak arguments, such as the extent of his practical experience—therefore, his judgment should not be questioned. As a result the worker leaves the discussion feeling angry, frustrated, and hostile towards the supervisor. It is also possible that the worker wants to accept the criticism in good faith, but rebels at the injustice of it all. Similarly, it is unjust to confront a client with an evaluation unless the material has been previously discussed. The fact that the material has been discussed before does not ensure agreement nor does it avoid all hostile feelings, but it does create a good opportunity for the client to ventilate feelings that can then be dealt with therapeutically. Thus, this method of handling the situation would appear to be professionally sound.

The following case histories illustrate how some rejections were handled:

Case 1.

Mr and Mrs A, a young couple fairly prominent in activities important to the agency, sought to adopt their first child. They already had one natural child five years of age. Both were highly intelligent, well-educated persons, who chaired discussion groups dealing with family life and its responsibilities. Intellectually, they presented a normal social history and avoided getting involved in any controversy. Problems that presented themselves were always passed off as being resolved and of no consequence. Mrs A had had a rather restrictive, disciplined childhood but denied any implications of rebellion against control. Throughout the interviews the worker had the feeling that although they were quite co-operative, the applicants were intellectually reserved and were keeping at a distance from the material they were presenting. They seemed to have considerable difficulty in focusing on themselves or in discussing any emotional involvement between themselves and the material they brought out.

On a home visit the worker soon became aware that the mother had a great deal of difficulty restraining the five-year-old. He continually ran away from her, was disobedient and beyond her control. In desperation she resorted to bribing the boy with treats in order to keep him in the living room with them. Sensing the mother's embarrassing predicament, the worker finally suggested that it was all right for the child to leave. When the child left the room, the worker expressed his concern over Mrs A's lack of control and inability to set limits with the child. A discussion followed in which Mrs A became defensive about her handling of the child and insisted that he was never this way at any other time, the worker had caught her at an off-guard moment, and that something else must be wrong. She found it difficult to acknowledge that this was anything more than an unusual situation, and rebelled at the thought that her son probably behaved in this manner more frequently than she realized.

Out of the ensuing discussion a rationale was developed for the need of psychological testing, to which Mrs A reluctantly agreed. As it happened, the boy refused to take the examination, and the psychologist reported his impression of an extremely aggressive, negativistic young child who resisted the tests despite the parents' pressure on him to do so, even becoming openly angry with him. In many ways he thought the parents had tried to force the boy to take the tests, but that he had successfully resisted them.

On the basis of this report, the parents were again seen for several interviews, at which time the material was reviewed and the findings frankly discussed. At first they were hostile and critical of the agency, the worker, the psychologist, and anybody else involved in the study. They came fortified with books on the latest child care methods to prove that what they were doing in the permissive handling of the child was condoned by all the authorities and that what the worker was saying was wrong. It was repeatedly pointed out that their son's behaviour was in direct relation to the way they handled him and that their own resistance to recognizing these negative qualities made it necessary for the agency to request a withdrawal of their application.

Slowly, in the harangue that followed, the parents began to see that their own behaviour at the moment was not appropriate and that in their desire to justify their position they were avoiding looking into themselves for validation of the worker's observations. Mrs A finally acknowledged that she did feel anxious and inadequate as a mother and that this was something for which she had not been prepared in her own home. Considerable hostility and anxiety were expressed about her own background, and from this point on she was able to concede weaknesses, deficiencies, and 'blind spots'. She brought out how difficult it is to raise a child these days with all kinds of conflicting ideas and opinions from experts and at one point turned angrily towards her husband and indicated that he had not been as much help and support to her as he could have been.

The discussion then became a less heated and more earnest account of a growing awareness of their difficulties, about which they had built an effective wall between themselves. The husband began to see that he also was involved in this conflict and by his withdrawal was condoning what was going on. Towards the end of the last interview they were exploring ways to get help and expressed appreciation to the worker for having understood their hostility rather than rejecting them without an explanation.

In reviewing this case one could conclude that the A's wanted the worker to reject them without any explanation so they could maintain their convictions and justify the way they handled their son. If this had been done, the worker would not have had the opportunity of helping them to understand better their relationship to the child. It also would have been easy to assume that this couple was much too rigid and well defended to attempt an exploration of their personalities. In addition, since the focal point was the behaviour of the child, what would prevent the parents from projecting their hostility onto him? Although these are certainly valid reasons for evaluating a case such as this carefully, they still do not obviate the need for interpretive interviews based on the actual reasons for rejection.

Case 2.

Mr and Mrs B, a young couple who had been married for ten years without a pregnancy, applied to the agency for adoption. The couple had undergone extensive medical examinations, and all reports were negative regarding Mrs B's fertility. The physician also noted that the wife was a tense, high-strung individual prone to gastric upsets when she was under pressure. In the initial screening interview the couple appeared immature because of their juvenile attire but, in general, seemed to show appropriate interest in the adoption process. In the subsequent interviews, the worker became aware that the B's had not seriously discussed the effect a child would have upon their lives and also noted their lack of financial preparation. The husband earned a good income—about $10,000 a year—and yet they had less than $100 in savings in addition to a huge mortgage and other fairly large debts. Mrs B was difficult to interview because of her defensiveness and anticipation of rejection whenever her adequacy as a potential mother seemed to be questioned. The fact that she reacted defensively even in non threatening areas helped the worker to recognize how delicately he would have to handle any questioning of this woman's adequacy.

To help the couple to understand better their lack of readiness for a child, the worker felt that it was necessary for them to learn more about their weaknesses and current limitations as potential parents. Without going further into the couple's background it seemed to be impossible to explain to them why they would not be acceptable to the agency as adoptive applicants. The worker arranged for separate interviews with the couple and proceeded to get the necessary background data.

Mrs B said she had had a rather unhappy childhood because her parents did not get along well. In particular she complained about the lack of communication between them. She also felt that there were no open signs of affection for her and her siblings. The worker wondered what effect her background had upon her, which helped Mrs B bring out her own discomfort about expressing affection and love openly. Mrs B felt that it would be difficult for her to hug and kiss a child if other people were around for fear of what they might think. She considered herself a rather shy and inhibited young girl who had been attracted to her husband when he was a 'big man on the campus' and because he did not seem to make too many demands upon her. This discussion of her background seemed to put considerable stress upon Mrs B and resulted in red blotches appearing on her face and neck. The worker mentioned this reaction, and Mrs B acknowledged that she became physically upset when under pressure. She immediately became defensive and stated that her nervousness would quickly disappear if she only had a child.

Exploring this idea further, Mrs B admitted that she and her husband had not done much thinking about the effect a child would have on them. When the worker noted that the same kind of situation made her unhappy with her parents' marriage, Mrs B quietly recognized that this was of deep concern to her. She quickly recovered, however, and told the worker that she felt she was revealing too much about herself and that further discussion of her personality would result in a negative attitude by the agency. Gradually the worker helped Mrs B to see that even if the agency came up with a negative decision regarding their eligibility as adoptive parents, she might learn enough about herself so that she could get some professional help with her difficulties.

In the interview with the husband, the worker noted that he had little sympathy for his wife's nervousness and regarded it as being of no significance. He seemed to be more interested in discussing his hobby as a sports car racer and justified his unconcern for his wife's nervousness by saying that if she could race cars at high speeds then she could hardly be a nervous person, since this sport requires 'guts'. His background was essentially normal, with evidence of some indulgence by his parents. He was drawn to his wife as a rather shy sort of person who did not make many demands upon him.

It was difficult to get a clear picture of their marital situation, but it did become evident that there was not a great deal of sharing or communication between the two. Mr B seemed to be less interested in the adoption than his wife and could only explain his interest in it by saying that this seemed to be the thing to do. The worker told him of the agency's many reservations about continuing with their application because of their lack of planning for a child, their limited savings in view of his good earnings, and the evidence of some serious underlying problems in their marriage that needed to be resolved before they should consider bringing a child into the family.

In the joint interview with the couple, the worker indicated that he wanted to discuss their case with the adoption committee, but that in all likelihood they would confirm his findings and would probably encourage the couple not to continue with the adoptive application but to seek professional help for themselves. At first the B's were hostile to the suggestion that they needed help in solving their personal difficulties. During the same interview it became apparent that Mrs B was troubled over her husband's lack of concern for her nervousness and general unhappiness. Apparently this was one of the few times it had been brought out in open discussion between them. The worker used this as *prima facie* evidence of the lack of communication between them. He warned them that this problem could only become more complicated by the introduction of a child into their home. At this point the couple seemed to be more willing to accept referral to a family service agency and indicated they would do so if the adoption committee supported the worker's findings.

The adoption committee did indeed support the worker's findings and recommendations and the B's were so informed. At the time of the telephone call Mrs B told the worker that she had already made application to a family service agency and intended to obtain help for herself and her husband.

In this situation it became obvious quite early that the couple should not be encouraged to follow through with their application process. It might be questioned whether it would have been better to tell the couple immediately that they were not fit candidates rather than spend three more interviews with them. It was the worker's judgement, however, that rejection would have been exceedingly difficult for this couple to accept in view of their defensiveness, yet to have rejected them early would have been unfair. It could have started the familiar chain of events of a couple's going from adoption agency to adoption agency without anyone taking the time to explain why they were not suitable at this particular time in their lives. The worker was aware that the couple did have certain basic strengths in their marriage and thought that if they received professional help they might return later when they were better suited for the adoption of a child. Certainly three interviews seemed to be a good investment in helping this couple accept their referral to a family service agency, especially if it led to a stronger marriage and eventual adoption of a child.

Case 3.

Mr and Mrs C, a couple in their late 30s, already had a seven-year-old adopted boy who had originally been placed with them for foster care. They knew the child had a serious heart defect that necessitated some restriction of his physical activities. Neither parent had a high school education. The husband was closely tied to his immigrant family, especially to his mother, who had assumed all responsibility for management of the family after the father's death when the boy was fifteen. As a youth, for example, he was made to assist with the family washing and ironing, which he did without too much acknowledged rebellion. At the age of twenty-one, when he first showed some interest in girls, his mother would not permit him to attend any dances since she felt he was too young. He had to wait until he was twenty-five before he could attend a public dance, and then he had to go with his sister.

Mrs C also came from a deprived background in which her mother left her father, when she was about thirteen. She recalled being treated as a baby and resented this. She had wanted to continue in high school but was talked out of it by her family. They felt it was more important for her to get a job and earn money than to get an education. She prided herself on having won a scholarship and spoke with some bitterness about not having been allowed to continue.

Throughout the supervisory adoption period the worker noted that although the child seemed to be getting a great deal of love and affection, the mother seemed to have a need to hold him closer than was necessary. When an attempt was made to discuss this, Mrs C immediately became defensive and justified her attitude on the basis of the child's heart condition or else denied that any potential problem existed. Several other areas of restrictive child handling were noticed by the worker, but he soon became discouraged from discussing them with the couple because of their defensiveness, especially the mother's. Consequently, when the couple applied for a second child, they were asked to obtain a psychological study of the first child, to permit a fair evaluation of the situation for another child. The projective tests indicated that the boy was alert and intelligent. He seemed, however, to have many fears and morbid preoccupations. His speech was infantile and he was regarded as severely inhibited. On the basis of these findings and on the worker's observations of the couple's handling of him throughout the past year, the couple's application was rejected.

In this study the worker was apprehensive about dealing with the evidence for rejection and felt guilty about having approved the study in the first place. Nevertheless, an interview was held with the C's and the reasons for their rejection discussed with them. As the worker reported, this was as difficult for him as it was for the clients. The couple, not being satisfied with meeting the worker, asked to speak to a member of the adoption committee. Their request was granted, and a member of the adoption committee and the worker met with them. Initially, the couple attempted to make the worker look incompetent by noting minor inconsistencies in statements he had made. They then tried to put the agency on the defensive by requesting reasons for the rejection. They were told that the reasons had already been discussed and were asked how they felt about it. They discussed their own feelings and expressed considerable anger against the agency for all the facts they could not understand or accept.

Their hostility was quietly acknowledged and the agency's purpose in placing children for adoption was emphasized—that is, the agency's prime function is to place children for adoption, so it is interested in placing as many children as possible. This statement was made for the purpose of removing the misconceptions and feelings held by many adoptive couples that since agencies have so few babies and so many applicants, they can afford to disregard the feelings of rejected couples. No doubt this was the case several years ago and may still be true in some areas, but in most parts of the country this is now changed; there has been no significant increase in the number of adoptive applicants, but there are many more babies available for placement. This couple was then told that the agency was seriously interested in helping them to understand the reasons for rejection in order that they might recognize the problem that existed between themselves and the first child, and also to help them to improve the situation so they could be considered for a second placement.

Patient and careful handling was the rule, with the adoption worker and committee member supporting and backing each other with a consistent approach. The hope that the C's would divide the adoption worker and the committee member was diminished, and they faced having to defend their position that nothing was wrong with the child or themselves. On this score the worker firmly but gently disagreed, offering excerpts from the psychological test and material from his supervisory adoptive period. Although naturally defensive at first, the couple began to relax when they received understanding for having gone too far in their protection of the child. This was seen as a natural outcome of their concern for his heart condition. Later, the same understanding was used in interpreting their strong desire to have the boy excel in those areas in which the mother had failed or had herself had strong drives for success. Both parents agreed that they felt deprived by the lack of a high school education and that they would not want their son to experience the same kind of handicaps. They acknowledged that their limited education was a factor in their concern about their son's academic progress, even though they had little to be concerned about, since he was a bright and alert youngster.

In an effort to get the C's to understand how their son's shyness and reticence had developed, their way of handling him was examined. By this time much of their hostility had subsided—particularly the wife's.

She was left more on her own as her husband began withdrawing from the conflict. Because of her defensiveness and the agency's lack of adequate material, this avenue had to be temporarily abandoned.

Another approach was used by having Mrs C reflect on her own expressed hostility towards her mother for treating her like a baby when she was a youngster. The worker's use of this social history information brought forth considerable hostility from Mrs C, towards her mother. Again, the worker expressed sympathy and acceptance of her anger. When Mrs C had finished, it was tactfully pointed out that her son may have feelings of rebellion against her similar to those she had towards her own mother. Previously she had acknowledged that her mother may not have had any awareness of what she was doing to her, so here, too, it was suggested that she might have a similar blind spot in not being able to see the same lack of awareness within herself. This idea was apparently difficult for her to accept for she changed the subject yet still asked what she could do about it. Until this time she had still been defending her position, but with less and less hostility. At this point she finally recognized that the problem was within herself and her husband, and she appeared eager to know what she could do about improving and rectifying it.

From then on the interview proceeded in a supportive and sympathetic manner. Mrs C experienced considerable frustration, but the worker could not give her any specific advice other than to ease up on the pressures a bit. It was also difficult for her to accept the fact that only when she fully understood and accepted what was being talked about and saw the problem much as the worker saw it would the solution become obvious to her. For her to try new methods of dealing with her child merely because they were suggested would result in failure. It was painful to her to acknowledge the need for making changes in her handling of her son, as this implied a recognition that some difficulty did exist between herself and the child. Towards the latter part of the interview Mr C acknowledged that he had been aware of his wife's tendency to exert greater pressure on the child than he would have done. With this in mind it was thought he might help her to see what was being explained. At the close of the interview Mrs C was no longer hostile but was somewhat confused as to how she could resolve these problems. She asked for continued help and was told it would be forthcoming.

The purpose in this case was to show the clients that a second child could not be placed with them because of the problem that existed with the first child. This purpose was accomplished. A second objective was to help the mother to achieve some understanding and insight into her child's behaviour. To what extent this was accomplished is less clear. It is known, however, that Mrs C is now less sure about her earlier manner of handling her son and is beginning to question the meaning of some of her actions in relationship to his behaviour. It is to be hoped that some of her confusion may ease the pressure and intensity with which she formerly carried out her convictions. If she becomes less secure about what she is doing, it is conceivable that she will not be able to follow through with the same force and vigour in carrying out her objectives as she had done before.

In reviewing the material on rejected applicants, it can be noted that rejection often appears to be more difficult when the family already has a child. One cannot help but feel that the intensity with which some of these couples carry out their demands for a second child is the result of their own insecurity and need to prove to themselves that they are adequate and competent parents. In conclusion, these points should be reiterated: It is important that the worker in an adoption agency be aware of the general attitude of his clients. He must realize that prospective parents are often anxious couples who come to the agency concerned not only over their inability to have children, but also fearful of the agency itself. They may be aware of and concerned over the possible detection of defects in their own personalities. Since most adoptive clients come to the agency in an anxious state, it is easy to see that rejection may prove a knotty problem, particularly if the caseworker attempts to explain the rejection. Yet there are sound reasons for telling prospective parents why they are being rejected. First, an explanation of the causes for rejection gives the couple an opportunity to understand themselves better and to correct their deficiencies. Second, a sincere, tactfully expressed explanation can result in a better feeling between the clients and the agency, which in turn can promote a better public image of the agency in the community. Finally, explaining the reason for rejection is just a part of good social work. It is the professional way of handling it.

Interpretation of a rejection requires skill and understanding, both in preparing the rejection and in explaining it to the clients. The worker must take care to discuss a couple's personality defects in an understanding and constructive manner. He does not have the right to shatter a client's defences in order to help the client know the truth about his weaknesses.

There are several principles that can make interpretation easier. The first of these centres on the meaning of interpretation. The worker's role in explaining rejection to his clients cannot be likened to that of the psychoanalyst who interprets deeply from the unconscious. Rather, for the explanation to be effective, he must rely upon interpreting only the material the client has brought out in interviews. He can share only those impressions for which he has substantiating data.

Finally, rejection should never come as a surprise to a couple. To ensure the clients' co-operation in the interview situation, it is wise for the worker to inform them at the outset that from time to time as he uncovers a problem area he will discuss it with them. For, unless the worker has previously explored every question he has with his clients, he is in no position to make a rejection.

13

UNDERSTANDING AND EVALUATING A FOSTER FAMILY'S CAPACITY TO MEET THE NEEDS OF AN INDIVIDUAL CHILD *

DRAZA KLINE

THE selection of a suitable foster home for a child would be a relatively simple business if foster children and foster parents were simple in their emotional make-up. But, since people are not simple, we are faced with the task of understanding the foster child and the foster family sufficiently to predict within reasonable limits how these complex human beings may affect each other in the close, continuous, interpersonal relationships of family life.

From the evaluation of past experience we have learned that many foster home placements, in homes in which the foster parents seemed to possess adequate parental capacities, failed because the child brought with him certain fixed patterns of unhealthy behaviour that did not respond to the care offered, and in some instances grew more severe. It is not enough for foster parents of such children to be capable of giving good parental care. In addition, in order to provide a corrective emotional experience, they must be able to withstand the emotional impact of the special problems the child may bring and the need he may have to get them to behave as his parents did; and they should be relatively free from the kinds of problems to which the child has a special sensitivity.

The foster parent who might give excellent care to one child may be so affected by a specific problem in another child that his behaviour is altered drastically. It has been a familiar but puzzling phenomenon to see a foster parent, after a substantial period of caring for a child, begin to behave towards the child, spouse, or other members of the family in ways that surprise and sometimes shock us. Often we not only did not anticipate this but, from our study, would not have believed it possible. We have tended to explain this phenomenon in various ways; the study

* Published in *The Social Service Review*, Vol. XXXIV, No. 2, June, 1960.

was inadequate and misleading; the foster parents are being adversely affected by other circumstances in their lives; and the like. While any of these explanations may be partly or wholly correct, there is another possibility that should be considered.

Are the problems which the child presents of a specific nature that reactivates in the foster parents problems from their own childhood which have been well covered over and dormant? Is it this reactivation of earlier problems that brings about the surprising and unstable behaviour? And does this changed behaviour reflect the foster parents' efforts to maintain emotional equilibrium under the impact of the internal stresses that have been stirred up? This is one of the problems requiring our special attention in study of children and foster parents.

It is not my intention to discuss the general content of studies of children or foster homes, or the general criteria for agency use of foster homes, since this information is available from many other sources. I will, instead, concentrate on describing a specific, theoretical approach to selecting an approved home for a particular child, its application in understanding the child and the foster parents, its use in predicting within reasonable limits the interpersonal interaction that might be expected between a child and a family, and its use in planning the help that may be needed by the family after placement.

One of the most elusive but essential areas of understanding the child is that which involves the quality and pattern of his behaviour in interpersonal relationships. His stereotyped symptoms are readily discovered in the study. A good study will reveal the child's overt symptoms, as well as his strengths in the major areas of development. For example, with an adequate study we are in a favourable position to know, among other things, that Johnny is a bright, attractive, hyperactive, eight-year-old boy who wets the bed, sometimes lies protectively, is good at baseball, is in his correct grade placement, but 'acts up' in school and had some trouble last year with a rather difficult teacher who did not understand his problems. His mother has been 'at her wits end' with him. She whips him for wetting the bed and 'it only gets worse.' We discuss Johnny's bed-wetting and lying, as well as his other characteristics, with the prospective foster parents. They accept and seem to understand all of this. And yet, the time comes when the foster mother tells us desperately that she is at the end of her rope with Johnny. His lying and his bed-wetting have grown worse. He is completely unresponsive and unco-operative. She has tried everything but 'he isn't satisfied' until she whips him. We then may well say to ourselves, reproachfully, 'This foster mother really can't tolerate Johnny's bed-wetting and lying, even though we prepared her ahead of time and she seemed very accepting and sympathetic.' As to the whipping, we probably are shocked. This is what his own mother did, and this is the worst possible way to handle enuresis when, as with Johnny, it is caused by a deep-seated fear of women. 'He might as well have remained in his own home for all of the corrective emotional experience he is getting here.'

This may well be somewhat the direction our thoughts will take. But let me suggest that we were not necessarily mistaken in thinking that the foster mother would be able to accept Johnny's symptoms of bed-wetting and lying and would try to work with us to find ways to help Johnny. There are some indications that our mistake was not what we think. The fact that the foster mother is now treating Johnny as his mother does not necessarily mean that she is like Johnny's mother. Like many other children in foster homes, this child appears to be the victim of a cruel fate, repetitiously experiencing the same kind of mishandling from one adult after another despite our best efforts to find him a good foster home. This circumstance should always be viewed with scepticism. In Johnny's case there are significant indications that it was not the symptoms the foster mother could not tolerate but something that Johnny was doing in his relationship with her, which she could not adequately comprehend or describe, which made the lying and bed-wetting *seem* unacceptable and which ensnared her into acting as his mother had.

The fact that a child's behaviour elicits the same kind of response from more than one adult should strongly suggest to us that the child is behaving purposefully, but unconsciously, in a way that elicits this kind of response because of his underlying need to recreate his early environment and pattern of relationships. In this instance, if we knew the nature and quality of Johnny's relationship with his mother, and, similarly, the details about his relationship with the teacher and with other adults, we could begin to get a picture of his patterns of behaviour in interpersonal relationships to use as a guide in evaluating the suitability of a particular foster home.

There are three questions that deserve careful attention: (1) What are the child's patterns of interpersonal relationship? (2) What are the vulnerable areas in the emotional make-up of the foster parents that may be reactivated by the particular relationship problems of a given child? (3) What are the vulnerable areas in the emotional make-up of the child that may be reactivated by the problems of the foster parents?

Dr Littner has described in detail the defence mechanism of the repetition of behaviour as a means of handling internal anxiety. We know that this mechanism may serve different purposes in different children or several different purposes in the same child. Exactly what the child tries to repeat depends on what has happened to him. The more disturbed he is, the less will he be able to respond realistically to the foster parents and others in his environment, and the more likely he will be to resort to handling emotional stress in the old ways.

If the foster parents, out of their own needs, behave towards him as his parents did, or if they are vulnerable to his manipulations and can be trapped into acting the role he sets for them, there will be no internal need for him to give up the repetition of disturbed ways of handling inner tensions. But if the foster parents do not fall into this trap, and if they maintain healthy ways of reacting, the child will gradually be strengthened by their help so that he will have more capacity to react realistically to what is going on and will find better ways to handle internal conflicts when they recur.

The foster child's early life with his parents is likely to include almost classical kinds of damaging experience: quarrelling parents, neglect, sexual trauma, premature burdens of responsibility and, uniformly, the culminating experience of being sent away from his parents. Consequently, the foster child, more often than not, is to some degree a disturbed child whose repertory of repetitive behaviour may be extensive.

Before selecting a foster home, it is essential for the worker to give careful attention to the child's characteristic ways of relating to others. The detailed history, including the child's early experiences and the quality of maternal care and his reactions to it, provides one source for predicting the kinds of expectations and reactions the child may have developed. A second source for testing the predictions made from the history is the child's current behaviour in interpersonal relationships within and outside his family.

The reactions of various adults to a particular child will tell us a good deal about him. In some instances a detailed history reveals that the child's disturbed and disturbing behaviour is restricted almost entirely to his relationships within his immediate family. When this is so, the problem is usually of relatively recent onset. The child who arouses the same quality of feeling in different adults under different conditions is a child who is not reacting just to the current external situation, but is reacting unrealistically, governed by internal mechanisms which he has developed as a way of mastering internal conflicts.

In general, the younger the child, the less fixed are the relationship patterns. However, a study of a fourteen-month-old girl can well illustrate two considerations mentioned earlier, that are pertinent to studies of children and foster parents: (1) the repetitive behaviour of the child in interpersonal relationships and (2) the sensitive areas in the foster parents which will exacerbate the problems of both foster parents and child.

A study of Ann at fourteen months of age revealed that she probably had already developed a significant neurotic pattern of relating to her mother which she would be likely to use in her future relationships with a mothering person. Ann's mother was an impulse-ridden teenager, who gave erratic, impulsive care to her baby. When the mother was absent or neglectful, the maternal grandmother took over Ann's care. When the mother and father were at home together, they quarrelled violently. At twelve months of age Ann had been removed from the parents' custody by court order following hospitalization for burns that resulted from physical neglect. She had been placed by the court in a nursery pending a foster-home plan. Ann was an alert and attractive child of normal intellectual and physical development. One might easily assume that her needs could be well met by warm, giving foster parents. However, with this kind of history, we would like to know, as nearly as possible, the exact outcome of the poor care that had been given. The child ate, slept, and behaved normally in every respect. The nurses at the nursery found her easy to care for and were fond of of her. The mother was too disturbed to give a coherent account of the early developmental history. However, there is a significant bit of information, often missing, which in this instance was available. In the course of the study, the nurses were asked how Ann behaved during her mother's visits. It was learned that the mother visited erratically. Ann often reacted, from the beginning of the nursery placement, by crying, refusing any direct contact with her mother, and showing a distinct preference for contact with the nurses. The mother felt rejected and visited less frequently. We then saw interpersonal behaviour that was no longer that of a child reacting to the mother's current behaviour, because during the visiting period the mother behaved benignly towards the child. Ann was not *unresponsive* to the mother's presence; she responded actively by rejecting her and turning to another mothering person. This suggested, at the time of the study, and was borne out in the subsequent placement, that she had already developed a pattern of turning away from the mothering person to another mother when she was frightened about the mother's feelings towards her.

It can be expected that, in the future, when she feels left out or rejected, regardless of how realistic or unrealistic her feeling may be, this pattern may be repeated. Since there are innumerable times each day in normal family life when a small child must and should be left out of the interests and activities that are inappropriate for her, there will be endless opportunities for such a reaction. When it occurs, the foster mother, naturally, will feel frustrated and bewildered. The foster mother will tell us that the child, at times for no reason at all, turns away and will have nothing to do with her. She seems to prefer Aunt Emma or the maid or even the dust mop. She 'takes to' almost anyone but the foster mother.

It is now clear that this vital piece of information about Ann's pattern of behaving in her relationship with her mother and the nurses is going to be of the utmost importance in selecting a foster home for her. While it cannot be predicted with certainty how she or any other child will behave with a foster parent, our job is to make a reasonable conjecture and to act within it in order to prevent, as far as possible, the miscarriage of the placement. Any foster parent will react with some discomfort to this kind of behaviour in a small child and will need help in understanding and handling it. But it will be important to avoid the selection of a foster mother who, because of some injurious experience of her own childhood, has a special sensitivity to rejection and a strong need for acceptance.

In addition to normal good mothering, a child with this kind of problem needs a foster mother who, with help, is able to ignore the defensive pattern of behaviour, and who will feel comfortable and not need to interfere when the child turns to someone else. If the child is not already too severely damaged, she will gradually respond to this change in emotional climate created by the foster mother with a corresponding change in her own behaviour. But if she is able to elicit from the foster mother the same feelings and the same kind of responses she aroused in the mother, her pattern of behaviour will be reinforced rather than changed and will bring her increasing rejection, which will in turn decrease her capacity to use good mothering as a corrective emotional experience.

If, by chance, this child is placed in a family in which the child's problem touches off a marked vulnerability to rejection, we may observe reactions in the foster mother that seem extreme and even irrational to us. The interaction between the two may cause the problem behaviour in each to mount, resulting in increasing tension in the foster mother.

She may handle this in various ways: by quiet withdrawal from the child, by inappropriate anger, by rejection, by oversolicitude and over-protection, or by other reactions, depending on what solutions are characteristic of her when she is under stress, and on the degree of painfulness of the early feelings that have been aroused.

If the problem is not too deep-seated and fixed, the foster mother may be able to use the help of the worker to understand how the child's behaviour comes from the earlier experience, and thus to feel less personally rejected by it. When simple explanation does not alleviate the problem, the caseworker who has established a strong, positive casework relationship with the foster mother may be able to point out to her that she is especially sensitive to the behaviour of the child, just as every adult carries with him some special sensitivity from child-hood. For a relatively healthy adult, this much insight and intellectual mastery may be enough to balance the emotional scales. It may bring from the foster mother some spontaneous associations, ventilation of feeling through recounting remembered experiences, and awareness of the connection between her earlier experience and her reactions to the child's problem. This insight should strengthen her capacity to relate more to the child's needs and to respond less in terms of the old painful memories, but it will not solve the problem permanently. The feelings will recur in different disguises under various conditions. It is the function of the ongoing casework process to relate the help that is given to the feeling needs as they arise rather than to expect them to disappear once they have been discussed. If the problem in the foster mother is too fixed and pervasive to be modified through casework help, we are faced with the necessity to evaluate the total relationship and its effects on the child's development in order to determine whether the placement should continue. Meantime, the foster mother is constant-ly faced with the question of her capacity to tolerate the stress that the problem creates in her and may initiate the request for the child's removal.

Another type of relationship problem seen in children placed in foster homes is that of the child who was either ignored and rejected by quarrelling parents or was used as an object for the discharge of feelings that belonged in the marital relationship. Among these children, we find those who have a pattern of promoting quarrels between others. It is not unknown to be told by a foster parent, 'Take the child away before our marriage breaks up', or words to that effect. But the study of the foster home had shown no evidence of a shaky marriage.

If our study of the child, which includes a careful exploration of family relationships, reveals a chronic pattern of disagreement between the parents, and the child has been drawn in as a protagonist for one or the other, we would be well advised to keep this in mind in selecting a foster home. We would want to look into the question of how the prospective foster parents resolved their own problems in regard to competition, jealousy, or envy. Although the marital relationship of foster parents may be stable and solid, either or both may be vulnerable to the manipulations of a child who has a need to promote quarrels. Some relevant questions are:

(1) Was there a history of divisive quarrelling between their own parents?
(2) Are there evidences of a need to become involved and take sides repeatedly in the quarrels of others?
(3) Is there a pattern of 'using' the advice or opinions of several people against each other?
(4) Are there evidences of severe conflict over competition or rigid denial of normal differences of opinion?

This information should be evaluated with awareness that a tendency to be caught in triangular situations is a common human reaction. In evaluating whether there is a special problem in this area, we need to establish whether the behaviour is repetitive or whether the emotional reactions to situations that occur are out of proportion to the facts. If so, we could expect these individuals to be especially vulnerable to the child's efforts to set them against each other.

For a child who has this kind of problem we would look especially for a couple who seem free from such problems, who share freely with each other, and who possess enough maturity to understand the child's need to behave in this way and to resist being drawn into it. Otherwise, they will be unable to help the child and the child's presence may prove destructive to them.

Another facet of this problem is seen in the little girl who has learned to handle her problems by seductive behaviour with a father figure. She will tend to relate in this way to new foster parents, and if either the foster mother or the foster father has conflicts that will be aroused by this relationship, the placement will damage the child and the foster parents.

An illustration of this is the placement of a teen-age girl who, at the age of two, had been seductively handled by her father while he assumed the mothering role after the mother deserted. Subsequently, the child reported sexual tampering by a foster father and by a man who lived in the neighbourhood of her next set of foster parents. Needless to say, she was a severely disturbed youngster whose pattern of relating to the father seductively was repeated with other men, precipitating repeated sexual experiences. After several years of institutional treatment she was again placed in a foster home. Under the stress of her re-placement, she regressed to the repetitive use of the old defence. She wooed the foster father, undressed seductively in his presence, managed to spend many hours alone with him in his workshop and in accompanying him on errands. Despite many discussions of the exact pattern of the child's relationship problems and needs, the foster mother was unable to prevent the child from shutting her out and could not use help to find ways to make the child a part of the family. She reacted to the child's closeness to the foster father by withdrawing, leaving them alone to watch television, or sending them on errands together. The child and the foster father both became frightened by the increasingly seductive relationship thus being nurtured.

While it is clear that the problems of both foster father and foster mother were activated by the child's behaviour, for present purposes I will discuss only the foster mother's emotional make-up, which made her especially vulnerable to this type of problem.

The study revealed that the foster mother had lost her own mother when she was only two years old and that she was close to her father, who remarried when she was six years old. Her discussion of her step-mother indicated that she had maintained a conforming, compliant, satisfactory, but emotionally distant, relationship with her all of her life. The absence of real emotional content in the foster mother's discussion of her stepmother, her dispassionate 'all was well' attitude suggested that 'all was not well'. Even from this scant information, it can be deduced that this applicant had considerable conflict about the relationship between her father and stepmother and about her own place in their lives. The normal child, at the stage of development of this foster mother when her mother died and father remarried, is unconsciously jealous of the relationship between the parents and wants to separate them, and consequently feels guilty about her wish. She solves this, also unconsciously, by her identification with a good mother whose acceptance of her reduces both her guilt and competition. After a child has been hurt by the loss of the natural mother and consequently has been closer to the father than she would otherwise have been, the stepmother seems to be a real interloper, and the difficulty of solving the conflict over the jealousy and wish to separate the parents, as well as consequent guilt, is greatly augmented. Had this historical information been evaluated from this point of view, the foster mother's current distant attitude towards the stepmother would have suggested that the conflict had not been resolved and that the foster mother would be exceedingly vulnerable to the presence of a seductive teen-age girl in the family, and perhaps to any teen-age girl. Her need to remain aloof from the relationship between her husband and the child can now be seen as a continuance of an early childhood pattern of solving jealous feelings which were frightening and intolerable. Since residual difficulties from this stage of development are not uncommon, we might ask what would happen if a younger child were placed in such a home.

Any child, regardless of age, who had not made a healthy resolution of oedipal problems would not get along well in this foster home, but a younger child, relatively free from the need to act out competition with the mother, would probably do well. However, since the length of time that a child will need a placement may be unpredictable, we would need to anticipate that, if the child remained in the home, with the onset of adolescence some problems would arise over and beyond the usual ones. It is especially important for the foster mother with this kind of problem to have continuity of relationship with one caseworker over a long period of time. It can be predicted from the history that the characteristics of the relationship with the stepmother may be repeated with a woman caseworker. The worker's awareness of this makes it possible for her to react therapeutically to the foster mother's tendency to create a smooth but distant, non-sharing relationship. Through this relationship and the caseworker's encouraging and supportive attitudes towards the marital relationship, some modification may be achieved in the foster mother's feelings towards mother figures and in her own self-esteem as a wife and mother. Additionally, the foster mother may be better able to use the needed help after a long-established relationship with the caseworker and be better able to work through the problems after an established, meaningful, maternal relationship with the child.

Sexual acting-out of any kind, as a means of relating to others, regardless of the age of the child, is especially difficult for foster parents to accept. While it is a disturbed means of relating to others, it is also an overt symptom which is socially unacceptable, and thus foster parents are in a position to evaluate with us, in advance, whether the child's problem is one that they can accept and work with. The foster parent who cannot tolerate this kind of problem usually tells us so quickly. But there is also a need for careful, differential evaluation of foster parents who verbalize acceptance of sexual problems, since, in our society, such acceptance is unusual, and non-acceptance is a more normal consequence of our taboos. Therefore, we look closely at the reasons for the accepting attitude. If it represents licence, over-permissiveness, or in any way is a solution for an existing sexual conflict within the foster parent, it will have no corrective value for the child. On the contrary, it will confirm for him this method of handling problems. The only foster parent who can meet the needs of the chronically sexually acting-out child is one who has experienced and been conscious of sexual conflicts which he has resolved and, therefore, he needs neither to repress them nor to act them out. It would be more realistic, I think, to consider institutional treatment for children who handle their problems in this way rather than to expect that effective foster home placements, in any significant numbers, can be developed.

A somewhat different type of problem emerges when we consider the vulnerable areas in the emotional make-up of the child that may be reactivated or perpetuated by the problems of the foster parents. It is a well-known principle that, in order to provide a corrective experience for a child, we avoid as far as possible exposing him to experiences similar to earlier experiences that were, in the context of the earlier relationships, detrimental to him. While, in most instances, duplication of gross problems is easy to avoid, there are instances in which we may unwittingly duplicate an earlier experience. A most common example is that of the child who is especially sensitive to depressive reactions in adults as a result of experiencing them with his own mother at an early critical period in his life. This child will have a more troubled reaction to depressions in the foster parents than will other children. Interestingly enough, diagnostic studies of foster mothers and of mothers of foster children reveal that depressive reactions are fairly common in both groups. If possible, we should avoid using a depressive foster parent for a child who has been especially sensitized to depression while still too young to understand or master the feeling of emptiness and isolation caused by the mother's withdrawal.

The problem of providing a corrective emotional experience for the severely withdrawn child who shows a marked need for emotional distance in relationships may well perplex us. The foster parent who can tolerate the withdrawn child is usually one who has a similar problem and thus appears wholly unsuitable to provide the child with the warm and close relationship which he seems to need. However, for the latency age child of this type, we need to weigh the available alternatives and define our long-term treatment objectives. While we may think of foster parents who are somewhat impersonal and distant and are defended against close, warm, interpersonal relationships as unsuitable for such a child, there are other factors to consider: foster parents who have a capacity and need for close family relationships are usually frustrated and disappointed by the withdrawn child; their natural ways of relating may arouse anxiety in the child regarding his inability to please them, which will cause him to withdraw further or to find additional ways of expressing his anxiety. While intellectual understanding of the child's needs will help somewhat, such foster parents cannot identify emotionally with his need for emotional distance. The goals of treatment now need to be considered. If basic character change is the goal, the child will require intensive psychotherapy in conjunction with his placement. It would then be ideal if 'ideal' foster parents could be found, possessing capacity for warm, close relationships and that rare sensitivity that would enable them to relate to the child almost entirely in terms of his readiness and his changing needs. However, in the event that this rare home cannot be found for the child, it is not contraindicated to place him with foster parents who are more distant in their relationships. If the goal of treatment is limited, such foster parents, if stable, consistent, well-organized, and non-punitive, can provide for such a child a climate in which strengths can continue to develop and his defence in interpersonal relationships can be maintained to whatever extent he finds necessary. Once we accept the fact that a foster home, no matter how good, cannot by itself provide optimum rehabilitation for certain types of children, we can be more realistic in appraising the type of foster family that can meet the child's needs within these limited goals. If intensive individual treatment can be instituted for the child, living in this kind of foster home is not a serious handicap to him. The chances are very good that he will get from the therapist, friends, teachers, and others as much closeness and warmth as he is able to use. But, regardless of some of the limitations, he will be better off than in a home in which the relationship expectations are more than he can meet and in which his own limitations bring negative reactions from the foster parents.

For the withdrawn child of preschool age, as differentiated from the latency age child, we would want, and could likely find, foster parents who could give a close parental relationship to the child. First, unless he is psychotic, the child at this age is not likely to have fully crystallized defences against a warm, giving relationship. Second, because of his age, his need for physical and emotional closeness over a long period of time is so great that it is better to take a chance on the success of a placement than to hazard his development at this age in an emotionally unsuitable atmosphere. And finally, since the child is still at an age when the parent is customarily in a giving role, with relatively little expected from the child in return, we would be likely to find a foster parent who could provide warmth and closeness in the parental relationship without undue frustration.

Some specific problems commonly found in foster children have been considered to suggest an approach to uncovering and evaluating the wide range of problems in interpersonal relationshops. One cannot avoid the inseparable question of the emotional make-up of the foster parents and the importance of discovering their areas of emotional vulnerability. I would like now to discuss the latter subject somewhat more explicitly.

The foster-home study in all instances is intended to yield a picture of the family as individuals and as an interacting family group. If a home is approved, the study must reveal a family of good character, adequate intelligence, stable interpersonal relationships (especially in the marriage), reliable employment history of the husband, interest in and capacity to give good parental care to children, and capacity to work with the agency on behalf of the child and in his relationships with his parents. Within this broad frame of reference we try to learn about other significant areas such as the personalities of the applicants and their children, the attitudes and expectations in relation to each other and to prospective foster children, the nature of their relationship to their own parents and siblings (both currently and historically), the kinds of problems with which they can or cannot be comfortable, and the organization of daily life. From this study we try to derive some understanding of the kind of child the family can accept and work with. This question can be answered best if we are able to take a detailed personal history of both husband and wife. Our object is to determine how the applicants were affected by early experiences, both good and bad, and whether early conflicts that resulted from adverse experiences have been resolved or remain as potential sore spots in relationships with children.

Many objections have been raised to the detailed personal history as a part of the foster-home study. It has been held that applicants for foster-parenthood should not be asked for extensive history, that they do not see the rationale, that they must not be treated as clients applying for treatment (which, of course, they are not), that we should be able to evaluate from the current life situation and certain limited information about earlier relationships the applicant's readiness and suitability for foster parenthood. It is my impression that these objections usually stem more directly from reticence of the worker than from resistance of the applicants. In most instances, the applicant, in the context of a study, talks spontaneously and naturally about some aspects of his or her childhood experiences and family relationships, as well as present family and social relationships, not in response to questions focused on obtaining a chronological history, but in response to his own associations to subjects under discussion and to the worker's purposeful interest in following these associations and eliciting appropriate elaboration with comments or questions. It is self-evident that an adequate history cannot be obtained from foster parents through a question-and-answer method any more than in any other kind of casework interviewing. History must flow from natural associations and direction on the part of the interviewer.

In regard to the rationale for learning a great deal about our foster parents, it makes sense to most people that understanding of foster parents will help us understand what kind of child the family can be comfortable and successful with. However, whether from the discomfort of the applicant, the caseworker, or both, we find many gaps in the personal histories of foster-parent applicants. Our job is to learn how to gather significant information, within the limits of their feelings and ours, and how to evaluate accurately what we get. Applicants usually do not talk freely about experiences of which they are ashamed, or about painful experiences, unless there is some personal need to do so. The avoidance of specific areas of experience is often as meaningful as what is discussed, and, if it tells us nothing else, it tells us that there is a problem area. One applicant talks freely about her father, discusses both her positive and negative experiences and feelings in her relationship with him. She says nothing about her mother and in this way tells us that this relationship is fraught with anxiety.

When a study is approached as a means of understanding patterns of interpersonal relationships, threads of the pattern can usually be perceived running through the history obtained.

A small segment of the study of Mr and Mrs G. will illustrate the point. The G.s applied for a boy in response to publicity on the urgent need for foster homes for boys.

The G.s had two children, both girls, who were well regarded in the school and community. Mr G., when asked about the request for a boy, said his wife wanted a boy because they did not have a son of their own and he would go along with whatever she wanted. He was sure he had no preference in the matter. He was reticent about discussing his own childhood and gave a perfunctory and sterile account of his family life. He has a brother, three years his senior, who now lives in a distant city. They write to each other occasionally. His parents both died within the past few years. Their home life had been uneventful. (Although some applicants talk a great deal about their lives, what they say often adds up to only a meaningless picture. This reflects a degree of discomfort about the applicant's past life, which, in itself, is a danger signal, and it is imperative that we find some way of understanding him.) Mr G.s problems could be inferred from his employment history and in the quality of his current social relationships, about which he talked freely. He had been employed for sixteen years in the office of a large insurance company. While his income was adequate, it necessitated careful budgeting, and he was dissatisfied with his lack of substantial promotions and growth of income. He found his work somewhat dull, but he did not want to leave this job to seek another, as he was afraid another job might offer him less security. He described the head of his department as a man who 'played favourites', passing him over for promotion and choosing someone else on the basis of 'company politics'. He said, philosophically, that this was unfortunately true of big business and of life in general. He enjoyed being an active member of the male glee club in his church. The men met twice a week for practice. Between this and his family life he kept busy, had little time for other activities. He was a little sorry that his wife and daughters did not like fishing, as he would like to fish on weekends. Perhaps a foster son would enjoy this sport. When asked about other fishing companions, he said he did not like the men at work well enough for this and he did not know anyone at church or in the choir that he would want to ask.

When we look beneath the surface of the employment and social relations of this quiet, conforming, superficially stable man, we can see a great deal. He can neither move ahead nor give up his job; he is unable to make companionable relationships with other men; his participation in the male choir is an activity well designed for diluted, non-competitive relationships; he cannot compete actively on the job, and he sees the man in authority as omnipotent, unfair, and unreliable. He cannot leave the job because he sees all men in authority in the same light. Nowhere in his life is there any evidence of trust of other men or confidence in his own masculinity. It is not surprising that a year after a four-year-old boy was placed with the family they asked for the child's removal and the foster father confessed to the worker that he 'couldn't help disliking the child even though he was a nice enough little boy'. He confirmed his feelings, saying angrily that when he took the child to the bathroom in the middle of the night he 'felt like flushing him down the toilet'. The presence of a male child stirred up all the angry feelings that clearly lay beneath his distance from men, his distrust, his inability to compete, all of which must have derived from his childhood experiences and relationship with his own family. It is needless to point out that hindsight should not be necessary to show that this foster father would not be able to meet the needs of a little boy. A correct evaluation of the meaning of the information we obtain in our studies is necessary for the effective use of the foster home.

It is possible to pass over a history of employment, social relationships, and interests without learning anything significant about the applicant. These areas are a rich potential source for understanding the quality and patterns of relationships, the nature of existing problems, and what these might mean to a foster child. As was stated earlier, however, the surest basis for prediction is a study that includes both a detailed history of childhood experiences and of current functioning in various important relationships. We would like to have more information regarding childhood relationships and experiences than was available in the study of Mr G., as a basis for understanding the strengths, problems, and needs of foster parents, but when we are unable to get it we have the choice of ignoring the available information, and running serious risks, or examining it closely for its possible meaning and drawing reasonable inferences from it.

There is one other question that arises so frequently that it merits special attention. Does the specific request in regard to the sex of a child always have specific meaning?

The more mature and free from conflict both foster parents are, the less difficulty they will have in accepting a child of either sex. In general, mature foster parents are usually willing to accept either a boy or a girl, provided sleeping arrangements are suitable. At the other extreme, some applicants request a child of a given sex entirely out of an unconscious need to make restitution and to prove that they were not injurious to a sibling or a deceased child of this sex. When this is the case, the study will usually reveal deep-seated disturbances in the applicant that contraindicate foster parenthood. However, somewhere between these two extremes, there are many adequate foster parents who specifically request a boy or a girl. Usually they are less comfortable with one than the other, although they may not admit it even to themselves, and may give various reality reasons for the choice. For some people the sex of the child may be the problem to which they are vulnerable. Their discomfort with a child of a given sex derives from a special problem in their own childhood experience with a parent, or sibling, or both, and they choose to realize their parental capacities through the care of a child with whom they feel comfortable. We need to treat the foster parent's request with full respect for its potential meaning, just as we treat other significant information obtained in the study. If we raise a question about the applicants' willingness to care for a boy when they have requested a girl, or vice versa, we should do so with awareness of the meaning of our request and of the risks involved and, as in all placements, should be ready to give the additional help that is needed by the foster parent when we place a child who, in some measure, represents a counterpart of his own problems.

This paper has considered in detail some of the most common relationship factors that play an important role in what Dr Littner has referred to as the scientific matching of children and foster parents. This is intended, in no sense, as an exhaustive examination of the factors that are pertinent in selecting a foster home for a child, but, rather, as suggestive of an approach that promises to yield more predictable results than those we have been able to achieve with less refined methods in the past.

As stated earlier, our objective in providing foster-family care for the emotionally injured child is to provide a stable foster home environment that promotes the child's healthy development and corrects his early injuries. To do this we must provide relationships with adults which not only do not repeat the child's earlier injurious experiences, but which successfully intervene in and render unnecessary the repetitive use of pathological patterns of relating to adults. The more precise our understanding of the child and of the foster parents, the better we are able to select the most nearly suitable foster home and to provide the needed help after the placement.

14

SOME THOUGHTS ABOUT DYING*

MARGARET E. BURNETT

IN talking about a subject as incomprehensible yet as inevitable as death, one is reminded of the little boy who went to his grandmother and said, 'Granny, daddy said that all old women over sixty-five should be killed. Does that mean you?' We all have so many powerful and conflicting ideas about death that I think it sometimes makes it hard to work with patients who are dying. It is our difficulties and not the patient's that obstruct our view and most of us are so frightened that we want to run away. To overcome this we must try to look at the problem objectively, and then the intangible fear of death seems to be eased. It is in the hope of doing this that I have tried to analyze some of the fears of death which I have encountered. As a result I have become increasingly aware of the fact that the patients' fears of death are the result of their fears of life. It is when we realize this fact that it seems possible to help patients constructively.

Death is the only event in life that we go through entirely alone and with no real knowledge of where we are going. It is the very essence of loneliness, and the problem we are coping with becomes the problem of removing the poignancy of loneliness. One patient, Mrs A., was running away from the thought of her incurable cancerous condition because she was afraid of being alone and of doing anything alone. She had lived for many years always seeking the company of others and trying to lose herself in constant activity rather than admit that she was alone. When one tried to trace back the need for this, one found that as a child she had been of fairly low intelligence and bullied both at home and at school for her lack of achievement. Her parents had not tried to understand her; her teachers were punitive in their attitude; and other children treated her as different and made her a laughing-stock, forbidding her to join them in their games and their friendships. When she was nine years old her mother died and she went to live with

* Published in *The Almoner*, Vol. XI, No. 7, October, 1958.

her grandmother, and the rejection and isolation that she felt increased. In working with her, one had to go back to this original idea of being ostracized, and help her to relive it within the security of a relationship which took away the loneliness, and as this loneliness decreased, so also did her fears of death.

Another fear is that of a patient who thinks that death will take away whatever personality he or she has. Such patients are afraid of the nothingness where they will no longer exist. They cannot let go of life which has given them some tenuous sense of value.

This is a problem of helping patients to feel that they have an intrinsic value. It is because they fear that this value does not exist that they fight for it, trying to prove their worth to themselves. Miss B. had been brought up in a good working-class home. Her parents had always gone out to work in order to make the home materially comfortable. They slaved to achieve material standards and doted upon the daughter who was growing up. The mother gave her everything she could in the way of gifts; she organized her life for her so that she would not need to bear the burdens of life herself; and she tied her daughter firmly to her apron strings so that she would be safely protected from the hazards of the world. Miss B. grew up without any sense of her own personal strengths, and fought against this by trying to exert herself and prove herself. When she left school she got a job for herself and did well and felt she had her own life. But she lived at home, and on coming home each night the life that was hers seemed snuffed out like a candle. With the taste of liberty, the oppression of her mother's demands became more irksome and life was lived with this constant struggle for freedom and inability to break free. With the thought of death came the fear of the final annihilation of herself. The value about which she had never been sure seemed about to be lost in the blankness of death. When working with Miss B., one had to help her to win this struggle and free herself from her mother by giving her a relationship which was not possessive and encouraging her to grow into a knowledge of her own worth. As she found herself, the fears of losing herself diminished.

Then there is fear of the after-life. Some envisage a wrathful God who will tooth-comb through all the sins they have committed and the minor misdemeanours that loom so important. Mr C. was such a man. As he lay in bed, gradually succumbing to his chronic bronchitis and the general deterioration of his physical organs, he was continually oppressed by the thought of the evil of his life. He saw God as a punitive Being who would make him suffer for everything he had done. Mr C. had lived all his life under this constant fear of punishment. As a child he had been one of a fairly large family. They were poor and his mother was worn out by childbearing and by the struggle with life which a dissolute husband brought. Mr C. was constantly knocked around and punished heavily for every childish crime. It was as though his father gained satisfaction through making the children suffer, and this was the picture Mr C. had of any father, earthly or heavenly. Again, in working with this patient, one had to help him through these early fears by talking about them and helping him realize that they were a result of childhood experiences and no longer relevant.

Perhaps the most difficult fear of all to alleviate is that of the more mature persons who cannot bear the idea of the suffering their death will cause to those whom they love. The wife, in facing death, thinks of her husband's grief, and the mother contemplates her children's deprivation. One can try to understand this by saying that this is an over-responsible attitude, and must derive from the need to feel indispensable, but this does not fully deal with the problem. We know that if anyone in life is practically indispensable it is the mother of developing children, and here we have a reality problem, for the children are likely to suffer if the mother dies. How can we then relieve such a patient, for her fear is based on reality and comes out of a maturity that can contemplate others' needs and not her own? I do not know the answer to this problem unless the only way that such people can face death is through a faith in God that will allow them to hand over the responsibility of the lives of those they love to God. This, I feel, is outside the scope of casework.

If, when working with patients, we can see death in its relation to life in this way, we ourselves will surely be more able to face the problems that arise, and so help constructively the patients in our care who are confronted by it.

COMMUNICATION WITH THE PATIENT*

HELEN M. LAMBRICK

Some time ago, I selected for a student the case of an old lady aged 77, with chronic bulbar palsy, a neurological condition making it impossible for her to speak, and very difficult to eat. She was referred by the medical staff who thought there was some kind of discharge problem and that she could not return to her own home but would have to live with a married daughter or be placed in an old people's home. The student went along to the ward and a most helpful house physician explained the medical position, and told her what he knew of the social situation. She thanked him and said she would go and see Mrs P. straight away—'Oh,' he said kindly, 'it would be a complete waste of your time to go and see her, she can't speak a word.' However, the student insisted and at once became aware of Mrs P.'s desperate need to communicate her feelings and wishes, and of her deep sense of frustration at being regarded as beyond communication because she could no longer speak. The student conveyed to Mrs P. her concern and her respect for her as a person and her wish to understand and share her problems, not only through the one-way medium of words but through the non-verbal language common to them both, the language of expression, gesture, posture, touch, silence. Mrs P. was able to write words and the student picked up the feeling tones from Mrs P.'s expression and affect as she handed her the notebook to read. She was able to recognize that Mrs P. had very mixed feelings about her daughters and that she was adamant that she did not want to live with either of them Mrs P.'s obvious emotion as she wrote her wish to return home to her lodger conveyed the strength of her relationship with him and her longing to be with him again. The interviews with Mrs P. took place over two or three days, and although the doctors were pressing for action the student never allowed her own feelings of being harassed to disturb the calm, unhurried atmosphere she created with Mrs P. Sub-

* Published in *The Almner*, Vol. XV, No. 7, October, 1962.

sequent interviews with Mrs P.'s daughters confirmed the impression of rivalry between them and strong resentment of the lodger and revealed mutual determination to exploit the present situation for their own ends. However, with the student's support, Mrs P. was enabled to withstand pressure from all sides and returned home to her lodger. The student visited them and was struck by the ways in which he showed his affection for Mrs P. and by her delighted and very feminine response to his remark—'Well, she may not be able to speak but she has very bonnie blue eyes.'

I have quoted from this case, which might have had such an unhappy outcome, at some length because it brought into consciousness for me the many-channel system of communication which exists between human beings, and what particularly heavy demands are made on the sensitivity, imagination, flexibility, self-awareness and self-discipline of all those who work with sick people and especially those whose main function is often described as 'just listening'. I think that perhaps the stage when we move from 'just listening' to really 'hearing' what our patients are saying to us is one of the most exciting milestones in our professional life—and 'hearing' involves so much more than our ears.

In considering the ways in which we 'hear' our patients and communicate with them, I am using Dr Ainslie Meares's four types of communication[1] as a starting point and will develop these in relation to casework in the medical setting. I will also be discussing some of the barriers to effective communication and some examples of the conscious and unconscious content of communication.

Dr Meares classifies the four main channels of communication as literal verbal communication, unverbalized phonation, extra-verbal communication, and non-verbal communication.

The first of these, literal verbal communication, is the straightforward 'communication of facts by the logical use of words'. This is the only channel of communication envisaged by the doctor who told the student she would be wasting her time if she went to see Mrs P. Even if this channel is open, we must never allow our attention to be diverted from other channels.

Unverbalized phonation is the term he uses to cover all the grunts and groans, ums and ahs, sighs and squeaks with which human beings communicate primitive ideas of love and hate, pain and fear, joy and sorrow. This is the language of the patient who is reacting to acute physical or psychic pain by regressing to an earlier phase of develop-

[1] Dr Ainslie Meares, 'Communication with the Patient,' *The Lancet*, London, Vol. I, No. 7126, March 26, 1960.

ment. Noisy weeping and moans of pain are everyday examples of this.

Extra-verbal communication is defined by Dr Meares as 'the communication of ideas conveyed by the implied meaning of words as distinct from the logical content of the words' and I think that this probably covers a good deal of the communication between worker and client. At its simplest this is 'reading between the lines' and at its most complex we must look at the unconscious communication between patient and analyst. Extra-verbal communication includes all the innuendoes, changes of stress given to words, voice tone, etc., by which people convey, consciously or unconsciously, that the spoken words have two different meanings—the logical meaning and the implied meaning. Extra-verbal communication cannot be seen apart from non-verbal communication as it is through the patient's expression, posture, gesture, etc., that he communicates his feelings and tells us what he is really saying to us. We are all familiar with the girl who says in dull, flat, cold tones, 'My mother's very nice. She's had a very hard time and I'm very grateful to her' and then her face lights up and her eyes become warm and affectionate as she says, 'But my brother, now there's someone I can really talk to.' The girl who said this to me this morning was almost certainly aware that I understood what she was saying because I had already picked up several earlier extra-verbal communications with which she was testing me out, but often our patients are not conscious of what they are communicating, and many of them are quite unused to expressing their fears and feelings and having their communications heard and understood, and may need considerable help from us to be able to do so comfortably. Few of them will be aware of this aspect of the social worker's function and therefore the responsibility for interpreting this and reaching out towards the client lies with us.

I think at this point we need to look at ways in which we do reach out towards our patient and at just what we want to be able to communicate to him to enable him to communicate with us. The core of our communication is that we care about him. We accept him, emotionally as well as intellectually. We see him as a person of worth and of dignity, however undignified he may feel his present situation to be—and people do feel very undignified with tubes and bottles extending from every orifice. We want him to know that we feel sympathy and compassion for him but that we believe he has resources, unsuspected perhaps by himself, for coping with his problems and that we are prepared to help him do this—until the end if need be. We want him to feel that he has our full attention and that we begin from where he is and move at his pace, prepared to go with him wherever he leads and that there are no roads too painful or too frightening for us to travel with him. Going at his pace may mean sitting in silence for long periods. It may mean spending six interviews talking about generalities, establishing the right climate for him to say in the middle of the seventh: 'sometimes I wonder if I'll ever go out of here alive.' Being where he is invariably means starting from his physical symptoms—recognizing signs of fatigue, pain, discomfort—awareness of immediate physical needs which can be met simply by pouring a drink, peeling an orange, filling a hot water bottle, closing a window—there are dozens of examples of how we reach out to our patients and communicate our concern for them and our understanding of something of what their illness means to them. I think perhaps the widest gulf in life is between sickness and health and one of which our patients are usually far more conscious than we ourselves, and any imaginative attempt to reach across this gulf appears to have a good deal of meaning for most patients and is a vital part of the development of the casework relationship in this setting.

Touch is another non-verbal means of communicating our concern for our patient and our wish to share his situation. I recently saw a young Spanish woman dying of kidney disease. She spoke little English and the family were planning to send her back to Spain to die. Before involving myself in these plans I wanted to make sure that this was what she wanted to do. I tried to convey to her through facial expression, tone of voice, simple words, etc., why I was seeing her and at the end of the interview felt I needed to know if we had understood each other. As I stood up to leave her I held out my hand which she grasped tightly between her own. This reassured me that she had understood that I wanted to help her and that she wanted me to go ahead with plans for her return home. Often the only way in which we can communicate our continued interest and concern to very sick patients is through touch, and a sensitive worker can always tell when this is appropriate or when it would be too threatening for an inhibited patient. Dying patients feel very lonely and I think they feel less isolated and already beyond this world if we can reach out to them quite literally. Patients whom we are seeing in the terminal stages of illness are usually people we have known for some time and I know from my own experience of working in a hospital where all my patients had cancer and many died during the two years I was there, that the illness and relationship often reach a stage where all that is needed is the comfort of physical presence and contact, even a few minutes each day has great meaning for very sick patients. Sometimes hand holding is not enough. A few weeks ago a young woman thousands of miles from her family was sitting up in bed behind the curtains waiting to go to the theatre for a radium implant. In the past four months she had faced the birth of her seventh child, a sudden hysterctomy, an emergency flight to England, radiotherapy treatment and the knowledge that she had cancer. I had seen her every day since her admission and she had been able to express a good deal of feeling about what had happened. However she was completely panic-stricken and revolted by the idea of the insertion of radium. I don't think I have ever seen anyone so obviously over-whelmed by terror. I sensed this had some deep unconscious meaning for her and before I had time to rationalize myself out of answering the desperate appeal in her eyes, found I had moved towards her and at the same moment she flung herself into my arms and I was able to 'contain' her there until the nurse came with the injection. There was no other way of meeting her deep primitive need and I was thankful I had not been prevented from recognizing and meeting this by funny ideas about 'not getting too emotionally involved'. We must be emotionally involved to do effective casework—the danger lies in our failure to move into an effective relationship with clients and when we are not aware of what is or is not happening within the relationship. Con-trolled emotional involvement[1]—which is not at all the same thing as being involved—is the heart of the casework relationship without which communication barely begins.

What are some of the other barriers to communication? Fear that the client is leading us, consciously or unconsciously, into dangerous waters; towards awkward questions about the diagnosis; discussion of death; or of sexual material; or of family relationship, reactivating unresolved conflicts of our own; anxiety and feelings of inadequacy that we cannot help our patient; inability to tolerate hostility expressed towards ourselves or the hospital; concern about our performance, self-consciousness because we are afraid that we are being overheard. In a word self concern when we are focusing on our own fears, feelings and needs instead of on our clients. Overcoming this barrier is a constant challenge to most of us and I think we all recognize the times when we have been particularly successful, or failed miserably.

When we do overcome the barriers and convey to the patient that we are free and willing to hear, what kind of things do they communicate to us, consciously and unconsciously, through all four channels of communication?

[1] For a full discussion of this see Felix P. Biestek, S.J., *The Casework Relationship*, The Loyola University Press, Illinois, 1957. English edition published by George Allen and Unwin, London.

In hospital we meet every day human beings who are 'facing conditions that are among the most elementally disturbing to mankind'—dependency, pain, mutilation with its threat to bodily integrity and previously well-established and successful patterns of adaptation and functioning, loss of self-esteem, loss of love, and above all, death itself. Our knowledge of personality growth and development and structure helps us to understand the extent of the threat of, for example, amputation of a limb to an immature self-absorbed, narcisstic woman—or of a colostomy to a rigid man, obsessed with the need for meticulous cleanliness. They may deny most strongly that they are the least bit worried, but in the very violence of the tone of voice in which they say this they communicate the depth of their fears and the amount of energy being used to maintain this defence against the acute anxiety aroused by this severe threat. It is in these feeling areas surrounding mutilation and death that we need to be most sensitive and alert for extra-verbal and non-verbal communication including awareness of involuntary non-verbal communication such as skin changes. For example, sweating, turning pale or blushing or trembling. A very striking example of this kind of involuntary physical communication of feeling, in this case fear, was described to me recently by a young patient who knows she is going to die soon. She was so terrified by the final noisy breathing of the dying woman in the next bed that she found herself suddenly and spontaneously vomiting. Very few patients in hospital express their fear of death to the medical and nursing staff by direct verbal communication, and if they did they would in most cases be subjected to such a barrage of reassurance that it would be a long time before they did it again. However, every social worker who works with sick people becomes familiar with the tentative extra-verbal means by which they test out our willingness to share their fears. For example, the patient who says: 'This has been a good year for roses' and then adds reflectively: 'I wonder what they will be like next year.' The young mother with leukaemia who tells me her child is being well looked after by her sister and says, 'Oh no, I've no worries on that score' and then when I ask on what score she does worry replies at once: 'getting better!' Some of these openings are quite heavily disguised and often quite unconscious or barely half conscious. Another patient with lung secondaries was telling me about her three-year-old son becoming very companionable, and said that just before she came back into hospital he found her crying and tried to comfort her, telling her she would soon be better. I asked her if she often felt like crying and she replied: 'It is hard to have to leave my child without seeing him grow up.' Some patients can never be as explicit as this but talk about death as a philosophical issue or as a happy release for some other patient, I think all these communications have to be picked up in the patient's terms and we have to be particularly sensitive to where he wants to go. I think he feels that once the fact that he is going to die is explicit between us he has passed the point of no return and he has to be very sure that we are not going to abandon him with his certain knowledge.

Patients who have undergone mutilating surgery invariably have deep feelings about this. The variation in intensity depends on their personality structure and the threat to their present way of living. A woman who sees her worth in terms of her body is going to be very threatened by a radical mastectomy. One woman communicated what surgery meant to her and her need for the worker's acceptance in spite of her damaged body by showing her first the mastectomy site and then the normal breast. Many patients communicate their loss of selfesteem and deep feelings about their damaged bodily integrity by the urgency with which they demand that we look at a scar, or at a colostomy, and the need to feel that they are accepted in spite of this. A colleague of mine worked for seven months with a retired gardener who could not speak following particularly disfiguring head and neck surgery. The interviews took the form of written communications on his part, a slow and painstaking procedure 'just exactly as if he were writing plant labels'. At first his communications were factual. She was very well aware of the non-verbal communication which enabled her to pick up the feeling tones and gradually—through her sensitive interpretations—he was enabled to write down his feelings and finally could express in the most violent language his anger towards the surgeons who had done this to him and towards the men in the ward who treated him as though he could neither hear nor understand because he could not speak. He repeatedly showed her his mutilated neck and the hole through which the saliva drained constantly and communicated his desperate need to be seen as a person of worth by writing long accounts of his successes as a gardener and as a pig breeder.

Patients facing death, or surgery, which to many is synonymous with death, often need to communicate to us feelings about their fulfilment of their role in life. Some are clearly seeing their illness as a punishment—like the man who saw leg amputation as just retribution for leaving his wife and child for eighteen months. Some are asking us for our reassurance and approval that they have fulfilled their role and can face whatever is to come more comfortably if they feel that we have understood and appreciated this and recognized what they feel is

achievement of at least some of their life goals. Patients often communicate the intensity of their feelings by telling us about their dreams
—often very frightening. Sometimes their meaning is clear to both
worker and patient, as in the case of the patient who described vividly
a dream in which three beautiful snow-white horses came galloping up
to her and said: 'We've come to take you away with us'. 'Oh no you
haven't' she shouted and ran away until she woke up in a cold sweat.

I have already made several references to silence, which is perhaps
one of the most potent forms of non-verbal communication and can
be an expression of any emotion from extreme hostility to mutual love.
In the hospital setting we are often working with patients who have
never dared to express their anger and hostility in words and have
lifelong patterns of communicating these feelings through the rather
safer channel of silence. Part of our function may well be to free them to
express their anger, whether it is against ourselves, our medical and
nursing colleagues, or their family, by interpreting the silence and
showing them that they do not damage us or the relationship if they
do so. Many patients however are not able to express hostility even as
overtly as through silence—which lays itself open to interpretation—
but instead use extra-verbal communication, often of a most subtle and
indirect kind. A very attractive middle-aged woman with many features
of an hysterical personality who had involved me a good deal in her
complicated affairs, smiled disarmingly at me and said sweetly: 'It must
make you feel very good to have your job and spend all day helping
people!' It would be very threatening and unwise to interpret this kind
of remark to the client as hostile but perhaps one kind of hostility we
should always be ready to recognize and interpret with the client is
that aroused by separation from us—whether the separation is because
it is appropriate to close the case, or because we are leaving the department or merely going on holiday—and we should give our clients time
and opportunity to express this hostility and not leave it until the last
possible moment, when it almost invariably arouses resentment. I
think this is particularly important in the hospital setting where so
much happens without warning or explanation and doctors change so
frequently. Similarly when a patient is transferred to us we can often
pick up his negative or at least mixed feelings about the change-over
through such remarks as: 'I wonder how Miss X is getting on. She was
someone who really understood'—and recognize with him that it often
is hard to accept a new worker and give him an opportunity to express
his feeling about this.

To return to silence: I think we must be particularly sensitive to the patient's use of silence to communicate that he is tired and wants us to go away, but is afraid to say this in so many words. If we have misinterpreted this he soon tells us either directly, or through his expression, or by immediately starting a long conversation in order to hold us with him. I think however it is essential to convey to our patients that we are prepared to share silence with them comfortably and that they do not feel they need to be discussing their problems and deep feelings the whole time we are with them, otherwise they may dread our arrival. This is particularly true of patients who are in hospital for many months and for whom regular contact with us has often more meaning than we realize. I think we need to guard against feeling guilty and uncomfortable about these interviews in which nothing seems to happen for weeks at a time. We must feel free to let the patient feel free to use us how he likes.

A whole paper could be devoted to illustrations and interpretations of the symbolic meaning of the presents we are given, a very common medium of communication in the hospital setting. These communications range from conventional expressions of thanks, through presents obviously expressing hostility, guilt, or the need to appease—like the three large boxes of chocolates left for me on three successive days by a man who had taken one look at a convalescent home to which I had sent him and returned to London on the next train—to the kind of present which is charged with unconscious meaning. For example, a colleague of mine was enabling one of her clients to free himself from the domination of his dead mother. He had strong transference feelings and communicated his guilt about these by sending her pound notes, one of which arrived with a mourning card inscribed 'In memory of my dear mother.'

A further illustration of the kind of subtle, advanced communication by every channel that can take place between a social worker and a patient is the case of an intelligent 34-year-old Irishman who recently died of kidney complications following T.B. I was supervising the student who worked with him for five months. His communications were almost entirely extra-verbal and so filled with unconscious meaning that it was not until she had been working with him for several weeks and had a clear picture of the dynamics of the family situation that we even began to hear what he was saying. At first it was difficult to understand his prolonged discussion of Irish politics, literature, and drama and we were puzzled by the amount of feeling which accompanied his words. Suddenly it became clear that he was using this medium to communicate his own feelings and attitudes to himself, and his family. He was equating Ireland's struggle to free herself from England with his own efforts to escape from a dominating over-protective mother. Then we began to perceive his lifelong problems of sexual identification and his strivings to strengthen the masculine side of his personality, culminating in marriage with a young, dependent girl needing the protection and guidance of a father—a marriage designed to meet their neurotic needs which was completely destroyed by his illness and dependency. He struggled to avoid his wife's anger and maintain his role despite increasing physical weakness but within the security of the casework relationship he was desperately seeking acceptance of what he felt to be his real self—the creative, sensitive person he longed to be—and which in the last few months he was allowed to be within this professional relationship. The caseworker saw support of the wife in an attempt to free her to give more to her husband as an equally important part of her function.

Space does not allow me to even begin to discuss this whole area of work with relatives with the aim of freeing them to communicate with patients. Nor have I been able to touch on the cultural factors in communication, especially in our work with middle-class clients, which raises problems for most of us. Nor have I attempted to discuss communications with sick children, which is a topic in itself.

In conclusion, I should like to restate the universally accepted premise that all human beings share a common need for relationship and communication with other human beings. My experience of working with patients in two English-speaking countries leads me to the tragic conclusion that in our culture at least, many people live most of their lives with a deep unsatisfied longing to be heard and understood and that the kind of communication which is perhaps only possible within a professional relationship in which the other person is free from personal (but not emotional) involvement is in itself a healing, growth-producing experience, however late in life this may occur.

THE END